The immense value within the attribute of attempting to never take you too seriously is something that my horrific experience of suffering a severe Traumatic Brain Injury (TBI) has confirmed. It is what it is and now I wish to invest much of my time on fun, friendship and fairness.

This is inspired by Carrie and Chels – always with me every step of the way – eternal love.

Jack Martindale

BATTLING A BRAIN INJURY

THE LIFE THAT JACK BUILT

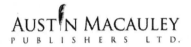

AUSTIN MACAULEY
PUBLISHERS LTD.

A CIP catalogue record for this title is available from the British
Library.

ISBN 978 178455 016 5

www.austinmacauley.com

First Published (2014)
Austin Macauley Publishers Ltd.
25 Canada Square
Canary Wharf
London
E14 5LB

Printed and bound in Great Britain

Preface

The process of writing my own subjective recollection of having a Traumatic Brain Injury (TBI) has been therapeutically cathartic. It is refreshing to have provided an existential account of my experience having a Brain Injury. There is a real paradox in talking about my accident; that of me being both immensely unlucky for it to have occurred yet terribly fortunate in the way that I have progressed since the first of January 2010. I've always loathed the ineptitude of the term, but I think for once, I can actually be justified in saying that my life was literally turned upside down. What has been crucial for me is learning to re-embrace life and overcome any feelings of isolation; as it is all too easy for me to feel ostracised in there being nobody who can fully comprehend my experience. A Brain Injury hardly goes towards the formation of any stereotypical pub conversation.

Seeming overindulgent in writing this is something that I am desperately trying to avoid. This process has been incredibly cleansing for me, as I feel that I have now fully reclaimed the ability for it to be completely my choice who I divulge my accident to. Another paradox in talking about my Brain Injury is it being a fantastic thing that I don't any longer feel an obligation to share my Brain Injury with new acquaintants, yet I can feel slight detachment from so many people being completely oblivious. Communication of my experience is now my optimum goal.

I am dramatically uncomfortable in potentially profiting from the horrific tragedy that I suffered. Five of us were injured by being involuntary struck by a passing car on the roadside— two of whom lost their lives. In spite of this, it has become increasingly clear that many of the gripes and difficulties that I've experienced are best described as things to which we can all relate; mine are only in an over exaggerated manner. My goal is for my unique experience of having a Brain Injury to be something that is worth sharing for mutual benefit.

Never thinking that worse cannot happen is perhaps the most invaluable lesson that I've learned; carpe diem. The last thing that I ever want to sound at all is self-righteous in anything that anything my experience may have seemed to have taught me. Being flexible about various life-paths occurring is a thing that I would always recommend.

1- All I really want To Do

Providing a worthy backdrop for relating the experience of suffering a Brian injury has not being easy. In short, (without wanting to sound more pompous than usual) it can be said that prior to my injury a good life was certainly had and has mercifully now returned. Defining yourself and your chosen lifestyle is hardly an easy task. With gratitude, it is possible to say that I certainly enjoyed living life; like I say, this fulfilment has thankfully come back to me. Some people unnecessarily never find it and probably never will.

Without wishing to sound like I am boosting my own esteem, I suppose that a 21st-century 'Likely Lad' is a description that I would have liked for myself. This said, 'laddish' is certainly not something that I ever at all was, but I liked to have a fun time. To me, nothing in life trumps a great party; throwing your own really is the cherry on the cake.

There really is no excuse for not attempting to enjoy life in the best possible way. In an outlandish way, this discourse has some elements parallel to a eulogy here. The major difference being that I clearly never died, so am under no obligation to talk of any life had by me using only hindsight. It seems sensible to live life with some plans that can be devised with foresight, but as I've learned the hard way, you can only really ever control the present situation to any extent. At times, giving too much thought to the future can only diminish your enjoyment of the moments that you find yourself experiencing. Attempting to live at a fair pace and not dying too young had always worked pretty well for me up until this point. The accident that I suffered caused me to inadvertently plummet from a high perch.

Disastrously I was hit by a car on the 1st of January 2010. The first term of my third year of university had just been completed and I was on track to earn a respectable degree over that summer. There is the contradiction of it being devastating that I inadvertently had to go through so much grief, although there was some relief that many of life's rites of passage had already been attained which relieves pressure.

Being struck by a car was less than 2 months after enjoying a fantastic 21st Birthday Party that I couldn't have imagined being more fun for me. (People leaving at dawn on a Tuesday after apologising for thinking that they have outstayed their welcome are always positive signs of a party's success!) Whatever petty gripes that may have been entertained by me are irrelevant in the grand scheme of things; I certainly knew how to enjoy myself. Dividing time between the University of York and a north-London life at home went down well with me.

Overall life had just gotten better for me since the tumultuous teen years had been passed. Never had I had (or indeed really been avidly in search of) a definitive idea of where my life would take me and this was something which had always seemed to afford me freedom. In the final year of my degree it felt as though you could be increasingly sure who would be your friends for life; this has even more so being confirmed to me now. There were very occasional times when envy was something that I had for people that could be definitive about what vocational path they would take. This didn't generally ever seem to matter a great deal to me most of the time, as I was just aiming to use my degree to get onto some sort of rewarding career. (It was lovely to be able to enjoy this innocence of youth...) Travelling had always been an ultimate pleasure of mine, so amalgamating this with fending for my existence had always appeared close to perfect.

Happy is certainly something that I was at the end of 2009 and although being confronted with death was not anticipated for many generations, I'd be satisfied to have concluded that I'd made my life eventful. On an academic and personal level, life for me was going pretty well. How circumstances can alter so rapidly.

In the early morning of New Year's Day 2010 my house door received a greeting which my dad can only describe as containing the "worst of worse" news for a parent. It was uniformly divulged by two police officers, that I was within the Royal London Hospital after having been hit by a car. Absolutely no further information was given; I can't even begin to imagine how this must feel. Circumstances were left most uncertain by the end of the communication. Whether I was in a critical condition or had merely broken a couple of bones was not at all clear. Of course things are perhaps all too easily said about being related circumstances once you have been given details of the situation, but I think my family could have been better prepared; not that there is really any correct way to relate tragic news. Dad, Mum and younger sister could then welcome in a New Year's Day by trudging across London in anticipation of learning what had happened to me. My parents assumed that the accident had occurred whilst I was in town, rather than somewhere within closer proximity to my home. Their journey was held up around Palmers Green, as a result of some serious accident, though of course the three were clueless that I was in any way connected with this cataclysm. With this in mind though, it sounds pretty credible of my mum to have said that one of her two greatest fears was confirmed upon entering the hospital. These dreads included me having being paralysed or having received a Brain Injury. The latter was soon established. An uncomfortable waiting game immediately began.

2- Here to Stay

Luckily I survived a catastrophic Brain Injury, albeit with severe brain damage. I was in a coma for nigh on 3 full months. This coma was by no means induced; waking up just never occurred throughout this period. As mentioned, two other friends died in consequence of the Road Traffic Accident and two others were also injured. I had the duality of tremendous grief on simultaneous accounts; both for me and my intrinsically close friends.

To use a ridiculously colloquial figure of speech in real terms, my life really had been lain out before me when I and my 4 friends were run into. No matter how much more time elapses, it will always strike me as rather dumbfounding as to how one vehicle managed to run into 5 completely disconnected passers-by on the pavement. As two lost their lives, nothing at all solely positive can ever be extracted from this upsetting ordeal. Being asked to feel grateful that worse didn't happen to me is important to recognise, though it can also be seen as selfish on account that two young ladies died.

Brain Injury still suffers an incredibly negative stigma. That being overturned would be a more than welcome relief. The intention now is to raise the profile of Brain Injury, as with rapid advancements in medical technology it is likely to be witnessed more commonly. The term would still almost make me shudder if I were not accustomed at dealing first-hand with the reality of it. I too was ignorant regarding what a Brain Injury actually encompasses. To use an egocentric cluster-of three, it can be said that prior to having a Brain Injury I was not unintelligent, unpopular or ugly. I don't think that I am any of these things now. Pretentiously it can be said alliteratively that right from coming around from my coma, my essential essence remained intact. Fortunately, despite the severity of my injury, I can still be articulate. A duty is something that I feel is now had by me to speak on behalf of the litany of Brain Injury victims, not able to currently express their thoughts at all coherently. I did face, like many other Brain Injury victims the double-whammy of having to recover from both physical and cognitive deficiencies.

The experience of initially recovering from a Brain Injury after having spent months in a coma really was surrealism to the extreme. I doubt whether many other people can vividly recollect contemplating being dead. I did, as it was seemingly the only viable explanation to me after being unconscious for what felt like an eternity.

Gravely poorly is something that I most certainly was. Thanks and gratitude cannot be overly-exaggerated on my part towards a certain surgeon in particular, Simon Holmes. The facial-reconstructive surgery he performed on my face, which exceeded over 30 separate pieces of titanium being permanently inserted, restored my face to how it looked previously. This is a remarkable feat that took place within the earliest days of this decade. There really is no time to waste upon deciding whether it is worthy to do this sort of surgical procedure. There was apparently much doubtful speculation from other hospital workers upon whether this was worthy surgery to undertake due to the chances of me coming around in any way to appreciate it being slim. Simon had the wisdom to realise that my recovery would be much harder from a physical and mental perspective if I continued to resemble Quasimodo. Unlike physicality, acknowledging any mental impairment is never an easy task without being confronted with a different appearance than you recognise. The swelling was so intense that my face looked vaguely reminiscent of a hamster's in structure for the remainder of 2010. Like many things, it is only upon recovering that you can really understand just how dishevelled everything was.

My Brain Injury is of the diffuse variety. I still go by an analogy voiced by a Nurse at the Royal London (the original hospital that I was stationed in between January and late April 2010) that a damaged Brain is akin to an office filing cabinet being turned upside down and its contents jumbled and scattered. The Brain, like those contents, needs to be reorganised, re-filed and rewired in the best way possible. It is no simple or straightforward task. Ending-up in a handicapped state, whilst experiencing an influx of incredibly new information being related to you puts your mind into shutdown. This is all too carelessly overlooked by many practitioners of medicine. At least I felt so anyway.

The precise location that resulted in the coma I was in after I succeeded being mown down, was by junction A406, just along from the Great Cambridge roundabout. This was after having travelled from spending New Year's 2010 festivities at the Brick House, a Club in Brick Lane, East London. I was with the same four close, tight-knit and old friends I had started the evening with – two boys and two girls. We had not had too much to drink at the Club because of the comparatively extortionate prices; we were all students after all. It was our intention to continue the celebration at one of the friend's house. Having walked from Arnos Grove Underground Station on the Piccadilly Line, we had reached Palmers Green when, circa 5 o'clock in the morning we were struck by a fast-moving car. This had mounted the pavement we were walking along as innocent pedestrians.

The driver as it transpires principally had the motive of guaranteeing that their car was not too badly damaged and consequentially evading any blame. I'm thankful that I have absolutely no recollection of this dismal period as I was momentarily left unconscious. The one remaining fully conscious friend dialled 999, for which I am eternally grateful for and have heartfelt sorrow that he had to witness this harrowing scene. Now I can't afford to even contemplate the likelihood of him not having been able to have called an ambulance when he did; every moment is precious when you're at death's door. Having heard of myself described as, "slender young man in a green puffer-jacket repetitively yelping." transports me straight to feeling that I'm in the third-person. Disturbed is how you feel at hearing a dramatic situation that you were part of described, whilst you were completely alienated from this entire process. Absolute carnage is probably the most accurate way to describe the scene of the accident.

I spent my 22nd year in hospitals and rehabilitative institutions. It was hardly the key to the door that I ever anticipated.

The time that I now recall from the Royal London was surrealism to the superlative. A bolt was soon inserted through my skull upon admittance to measure the pressure within my brain. Glad that I was completely unconscious at this point, as it makes me wince just thinking about it. Vague recollections from the Royal London that I have are just of a fantastic team of staff at the Harrison Ward at the Hospital. A considerable time was predictably taken by me, in terms of conceptualising the state that I had found myself in. It was only after coming to the Regional Neurological Rehabilitation Unit (RNRU) within the Homerton Hospital, in Hackney when things really started to gravitate truly for me. Up until that point, it had all just seemed nonsensical to the extreme. Recollections are reminiscent to having a nightmare. The difference between this and the standard deep-sleep, clearly being that you're not able to suddenly awake and put things back to normal.

This RNRU is where I was hospitalised between late April and early September 2010. The Homerton highlights to me how coming around from a coma is incredibly dissimilar to Hollywood's perception, where you suddenly just wake up and things soon go back to normal. (I assume normally after some revelation) In a nutshell, I can definitively say that I can only recount my entire experience as like something that only ever happens to OTHER people. Going back to January 2010, I scored a meagre 3 on the Glasgow Coma Index, which is the lowest score at which you can get and remain alive. I'm quite unsure what scoring two yet being dead means- an "active-dead" is not an expression with which I'm familiar!

Fortunately my parents, relatives and several medical staff kept a chronological diary of me coming out of a coma. It is incredible to read now. Amongst several little gems including me identifying photographs of images in French and saying "but you're too young to be my parents". (False flattery wasn't my aim here) Recollections of this period really reveal how far I had to go with my cognitive recovery. This was certainly not recognised by me at the time; I could only laugh when it was told to me that whilst an aunt was visiting my bedside at the Royal London: "these people are stupid, asking me to name what bloody dog is." To me, this seems to relate more to the circumstances of the situation that I found myself in, than any reduced mental capacity I may have had.

Identifying objects in French showed to some observers some albeit rather skewed logic still existed within me; a French language lesson would indeed have been my most recent recollection of being requested to name and identify objects. Understandable, I hope it is that could not accurately interpret the situation I had landed myself in. There was no context for me to use. I couldn't definitively say whether I was 10 or 100 years old.

The RNRU in Hackney was the optimum institution for me to go through this punitive experience. I think that overall it is a tale of two halves, where slow and steady wins the race. The practise really has illustrated the benefits of clichés and metaphors to me. On the one hand, there existed brilliant nurses and therapists who really gave invaluable deserved credit to their profession. On the other side there existed quite a few who have clearly placed themselves in the wrong vocation; I find this mystifying that they remain in the same ill-suited profession. You can but pity these uncouthly flawed individuals. Here there is the parable of me feeling at times like the innocent inmate of a prison. This does not tie in under any ethical philosophy of the criminal law that I'm familiar with. Any concerns that were entertained by me about my treatment could be rapidly dismissed on the grounds that I had endured a substantial Brain Injury. A doctor accurately informed my parents within the earliest days of being within the Royal London that as a pretty academic person, my recovery would be even harder, as I'd had more to lose.

Pre-morbid abilities are all too rapidly dismissed by professionals when relating anything to you. It was an incredibly alien situation for me, as fortunately I'd always been lucky in falling within the top ability grouping scholastically. There was a real reversal of fortune for me, as a considerable quantity of knowledgeable things had always seemed to go my way. If you believe in reincarnation, perhaps I was being punished for something in a previous life. From my perspective, this viewpoint is just too absurd in itself to ever entertain. What I most hated, was surrendering any privileges that I had earned to disconnected agents.

It's rather feeble that some individuals appeared to get a power trip out of instructing injured people. There existed wonderful medical staff based within the Homerton, though unfortunately human nature seems to overlook this when faced by crisis. Incredibly compromised is something that I certainly felt in the RNRU, which I unfortunately found to be an institution geared towards my purgative experience. Regardless of whether there was any necessity in doing so, being constantly analysed felt grossly invasive. Even closest relatives were no exception to this, given the amount of data on my cognition making matter of declarations suggesting things that did not sit well was not comfortable. It being concluded that you must have some lack of interpretation and acknowledgement of things that you have suffered is soul-destroying.

Part of my responses would have been down to cognitive confusion, although I maintain that the other side of it did merely due to part of me psychologically just not wanting to confront the bleak reality that I had found myself seemingly trapped within.

Incredibly insulting is how it can feel being required to display that I was aware of what had inflicted me. Communication difficulties in terms of my voice being recognisable is something that I clearly had and for a motor-mouth, this is far from easy. One thing that I tried to steer clear of concerning loving to voice opinions (in context, hopefully) was ranting about various things. Not only is ranting monotonous to be heard by any of the surrounding company, but from experience of listening to them I can conclude that they're often loaded with contradictions.

False niceness is something to which I incredibly object, especially when it is at times assumed that you are oblivious to what professionals are doing. Of course there are things which it is not always beneficial or effective for medics to communicate, but there is never an excuse to me to allow the ill to feel excluded. Living within this nightmare is something that I was never going to accept.

Having a Brain Injury gives countless the excuse to jeopardise any chance of you ever feeling like an equal. Many seem to feel that talking to someone with a Brain Injury gives them a license to say whatever they like as they cannot under any circumstance be held to account.

3- Heroes and Villains

In life you always seem to be confronted with an abundance of people who conduct themselves with some pre-eminence. Understanding what makes people like this is perplexing, as they are frequently without apparent significant intellect or aesthetic appeal. Concluding that they must be unaware that they are acting like this, or that they are just selfishly trying to simplify their existence are the only estimations that I've come to harbour.

In particular, I think that what antagonised me most was the superiority complex that encompassed significant numbers of nurses and doctors. It really is disgraceful, especially given that I've been lead to understand that there are sufficient efforts made to educate these people on how to divulge sensitive information.

Certainly the majority of medical staff are not inflicted with such a superiority complex, but there definitely exists a small proportion. Forgive the rhetorical question, but can a person acting so, really be anything but truly inferior, regardless of whatever pieces of paper they could wave around? A proportion of people seem to exist with some delusional facade. Perhaps that is being overly unsympathetic; insecurity is just a sign of inferiority that we as a society should strive to counter. Arrogance should always be viewed as abominable rather than acceptable.

Aloof people are only to be pitied themselves for their insecurity. With such people being allowed to tower above me in my hospitalised state, I really felt at times like I was on my own against the world.

Now I have certainly learned the hard way to appreciate the freedoms in life; as a lefty I hate having to sound right-wing in a populist way, but I absolutely can't abide blame-culture. Being fortunate in being from a fairly comfortable background (accepting that I probably am Middle Class was one of the hardest lessons of my teen-years) is what I've had to learn to accept. Particularly perhaps because first-generation middle-class is something that I would undoubtedly be officially labelled and class seems to remain to be the conductor of cultural nourishment.

Whilst it is a great thing for it to be conceded that society is undoubtedly more meritocratic in some ways than in past times, the propensity of the social class system in Britain seems to have ensured that many things have become vulgarised. Supposed taste is still dictated by the upper echelons of society and money can never purchase this in a way that can be culturally valued.

I resent how capitalist and thus unfair our society is, but you can't avoid but make the best of the cards you get dealt. It shouldn't be, but real choice IS still a luxury. Hopefully we'll naturally evolve out of this inequality, but I reckon that we've passed the days where Karl Marx's Communist Manifesto can be of any real assistance; it should come naturally from within. There is a failure had by me in terms of grasping how people remain comfortable with the unfairly competitive system currently in place. The disparities in wealth between different countries across the globe make this seem difficult within the foreseeable, though that shouldn't justify it in anybody's eye and I fail to see how it can ever be otherwise. Residing within a system so corrupt, it is impossible to see how people can afford to ever take themselves too seriously.

There is yet another paradox in that I found myself regressing back to a baby at the age of twenty-one. I fail to appreciate the irony. There is difficulty in having to relearn to do everything again, both cognitively and physically. Now I am fortunate, for it just to be the more tangible physical deficits for me to conquer. Contradictorily I just cannot overstate my gratitude for having been twenty-one at the time of my accident. Twenty-one really was in certain more shallow respects, the worst age for the accident to happen, as I was robbed of my natural twenty-second year of life. Yet I also had the fortuity of my brain still resembling plasticine in texture and therefore having a greater chance of recovery than somebody considerably older.

At least at the mature enough age of twenty-one the foundations were already grounded for my brain to rewire itself. Reassurance is something that I now have for never being too innocently naïve (i.e. boring) when the accident occurred. Oxymoronically I could say that I like to be a sensible hedonist, and going on with this I'll maintain that I'm an optimistic cynic. If saying this doesn't make me sound like too much of a complete prat.

In some ways, one of my greatest assets in recovery has been pride. I refuse to take no for an answer, yet attempt not to be deluded enough as to fail to see the intense recovery work I have to orchestrate for myself. Pride can be somewhat of a double edged sword for me though. I do not deny that at times it is the concept of feeling degraded that I have found most difficult to come to terms with, particularly when I compare my former self with now.

The situation that I've found myself within really does just reiterate how artificial many sociological constructions are; for example I've always believed that the gender divide is broadly exaggerated. It would be futile to deny that there is not any difference between males and females, only broadly speaking; we are all partly just androgynous specimens. Promising that I'm not just saying this to get in with ladies, I genuinely can say that vocalised misogyny is a thing that I find acutely embarrassing. It is rather cringeworthy, on the same spectrum as xenophobia, in terms of displaying and then trying to justify ignorance. (I think) If anything it can make me uncomfortably embarrassed to be of the male sex at times.

At times the shallowness of callous remarks ties in with people having a competitive attitude in terms of feeling like they have to prove themselves and score petty points off of one another. To me, it just seems that these people need to grow up a little bit, be a bit less infantile and get at least a vaguely mature viewpoint. As life just seems to me to be an entire grey area, nothing can feasibly be at all black and white, to use a convenient double entendre.

The danger of glamorising the past by creating some fabricated utopia must be recognised. All in all though, as said, my life was pretty hunky-dory; certainly in contrast to what I've unintentionally been through. Self recognition is an essential part of a healthy recovery, though I cannot help but feel that I have been treated in an Orwellian manner.

The fact that I'd never been familiar with many aspects of medical procedure should hardly be used as an excuse to allow anybody to be made to feel ignorant. The current practise of medicine does have the tendency to make one feel objectified. I think that this was particularly hard for me to deal with; although I can conclude that I tried to be a sociably affable person, I was nonetheless private.

I'm pretty sure that I wasn't ever overly conceited, I just believed that what information you share with others, should only be your choice until it directly affects others. It was pleasant to be renowned as rather elusive and this is hard to maintain when you feel that you are under a camera perpetually. There was a real change to my former lifestyle, where what I let others see of me, was my business and completely my choice. To me it had always seemed highly logical to live in a reserved manner; I feel that it always allows you power and control. We all surely should be adamant never to be pitied in any respect. Feeling that there must be people jealous of you is not what we feel comfortable admitting, but there is surely an element of us all in search of it. This is unless I'm just some abomination.

Now perhaps I can be paranoid. This is partly because I absolutely loathe being judged and told what to do; I'm not at all proud of this, though I doubt that this segregates me from an awful lot of people.

The hatred of being analysed that I have probably stems from being overly judgemental myself, which probably is based around some pop-psychology display of insecurity. Presumptions about your own characteristics are never a pleasant thing to be confronted with by outsiders; particularly ones you deem as lacking any authority to do so. This is why I always found it essential to try and build some positive rapport with therapists. Naturally assumptions are infuriating when you perceive them as being cast by people lacking the authority to do so productively.

At least I am able to recognise that many of my judgements are going to in fact be rather flawed. I deplore it when other people seem unable to recognise this in themselves. I've always attempted to be a winner to me in whatever I attempt, so a lot of my motivation comes from the thought of proving people I dislike wrong, as loathsome as this could make me sound. Part of my recovery has been founded on disproving people, as resigning myself to an inferior quality of life than I could have had is a thing that shall never be done by me in my lifetime.

Changes are things that I'm always willing to make, though if too much authority had been given by me to professionals, returning to my lifestyle so rapidly would have been unthinkable. You seem to need to allow authority to people in aspects of life, though for me, this is always through filtering out all of the people you do not get along with. The necessity of this cannot ever be underestimated to me; friendships with people you do like are what I equate as the thing I most value in life.

Freedom is something that was acutely missed by me when I was institutionalised. It is draining to constantly have to ask for permission for your human rights to be upheld. Independence is something that I felt that had been completely lost, as everything that I engaged in had to be run by other people, be it my parents or an authority figure. Overcoming this has been a slow and tiring process; psychological acceptance of my accident was the slowest process and perhaps too the longest of all of my problems to come-about. Once it has arisen to a level that is felt as complete by me I find it to be one of the most rewarding and empowering things.

4- Forever

Feeling that you have an exclusive relationship with another is precious and irretrievable once gone; I doubt that anybody in the world understood me better than one of the girls who lost their life in the accident. It felt like we knew one another intrinsically, though nevertheless I sensed it was the perfect relationship with somebody you love in terms of there ever being a sense of mystique, yet you know that you can trust the other implicitly. Ideally I felt that we were on the same wavelength, though different in many ways. Ironically there are always aspects of your own persona that the person you love is aware of that you fail to perceive. Beyond any sort of romantic interest I base all of my relationships with people on there being some area of mutual interest. This should be regardless of the disparity in your relationship; it was always painstakingly obvious to me which therapists seemed capable of doing this and those which did not.

What I perhaps most miss about my two friends who died, is that nobody could ever emulate putting me in enamoured hysterics in their way. Who is to say how we would have progressed as time passed; the fact that we were never allowed the opportunity of finding out for ourselves shall evermore be amongst the greatest regrets of mine. How differently life would be lived if we knew what was around the corner. Bereavement of the future was something that I initially suffered from upon accepting that I had suffered a Brain Injury.

You certainly can't do everything by the book as most things about life just aren't written down. Just making sure that there is somebody to always have a laugh with would be an epitaph of choice that I'd have. Not being able to open-up and understand people in the way that allows for wit, will surely make you end up all bitter and twisted, as melodramatic as this sounds. A close friend and I concluded recently that there is absolutely no harm in being twisted, provided that you're not bitter.

Humour is one of the elements of personality that I find vital; people who fail to interpret the satirical side of life always seem dense in lacking joviality. Bonds with people without humour can only ever serve a physical purpose and that cannot last that long. Of course there is the concept of there being a fine line between things you can laugh at and those which you would never dream of finding funny. Philosophy of spending a lifetime in pursuit of laughter has worked well so far. It is the knowledge that I have wasted thousands of anecdotes that I could never share with other people, who were founded on a bundle of jokes that would just not be found funny to anybody else that causes me greatest pain. With this, comes the realisation that there is a specific type of conversation that I'll never have again with anybody. This will always cause me discomfort, though going with clichés, scars can gradually fade.

Having friends encompassing diverse elements of the social sphere is something that I've always found crucial. It is good to morph into something of a chameleon, choosing which colour to turn, depending on your company. Being mates with a vast array of people has always been something that I've found essential. To me, only being friends with people who think in the same way as you, must just be a sign of narrow-mindedness and slight insecurity in that you seem simply in search of having your opinions validated. To me this can only be just a sign of weakness. This was another thing found especially awkward by me when I was under hospitalisation, as it's found reassuring by me to be enabled to select when and where to introduce friends to one another.

The person that I've loved and I would frequently rupture and could spend hours in hysterics about in-stories that would only ever be remotely funny to us. When feelings are too intense and the bond that you share is especially unique it seems to supersede anything deemed possible by the social construction of love that has ever been felt or understood by anybody before. This apparent distinctiveness can be blinding to us all and conveniently makes any rationality or logic become easily overridden. This is not meaning to undermine any of the impassioned feelings ever had by a person, but advocating just how complicated and inconsistent our emotions can always lead us to be, whist how certain they appear when experienced. The quantity towards which we mirror each other the way in which we view the world is something that shall never ever be understood. Exceptionality is a trick of relationships.

This is not to be solely methodological and formulaic about love, but it has to be accepted that there is some form of consistency in the chemical reactions that induce us to devote everything to another person. The beauty of this is that you fail to realise that when you're "head over heels". This would explain why enigma is the thing that I find most engaging and only increases attraction.

Being besotted equips you with emotions that I'd never have deemed to be possible. A safety is afforded to you by the feelings of love that you have and this is a real saviour to you as I certainly find that there is no fear quite like loneliness.

There were too many things that the connotations around to laugh at were found with the person that I've lost. I find that humour is the best way of bonding and this is 'conveniently' why I judge intelligence upon it at times; the worst thing is being required to explain jokes to people. What was so cherished by me, in a way that sadly can never be fully appreciated until it's gone, is feeling that you have a telepathic connection with another at times. Of course it must be accounted for that humour is a personalised thing, though you automatically feel downcast and perhaps awkward, having to explain what tickles you about a circumstance that you find hilarious. Bohemian is probably a label that I would nonsensically have quite enjoyed being called by anybody. Relaxed sufficiently and rich enough to be a true bohemian is something that I never at all was, unfortunately. My pretentious hat can be taken off now.

An immense amount of gratitude can be extracted from me at how far along the road of recovery I have come. I can now celebrate being able to "see the light at the end of the tunnel". (To employ yet another generic metaphor) I have been in love, which is why it is so important that I'm communicating this through writing, as I could never dream of saying that in first-person- not without having consumed any alcohol anyway. Of course I hope that I can love again; nothing else makes me feel freer. Part of attraction as well seems to stem from knowing that the feeling is mutual, if saying this doesn't emasculate me too much. It is harrowing for me to think of how this idea of being involved with the person that I've loved is so much in the perfect tense, as is my entire existence prior to the accident having occurred.

The element that I shall always feel most sorrowful for is the fact that I've lost the person that I could never truly feel unhappy or feel remotely ashamed of any of my history. That's what love is.

Confidence in my abilities is something that my parents have always thankfully instilled within me and it was empowering in guaranteeing my survival to know that if I ever died, I'd be losing a lot of love.

To deal with overcoming things, I detest the Americanised term "closure". What an ineptly crass load of rubbish that concept is. Suffering from amnesia upon coming out of a coma, I can't exacerbate upon how vulnerable and scared you feel not being able to recount certain stretches of your recent past. What is incredibly disconcerting is being made to feel like a disconnected stranger when confronted with episodes of your own past. I am so grateful that with the occasional prompt, all past memories have come back to me. Memories are a fundamentally personalised part of your interpretation of your identity and without them you feel incomplete.

They say that every time you try to remember imagery of something, you are basing your recollection on something you have dredged up previously. This has a domino effect on memories, it is therefore disconcerting for me to realise that the images of my friend will remain untainted and be eternally fresh.

It has always seemed important that I am careful not to delude myself by fabricating memory. The reason I cannot remember much of New Year 2010 I think, is part of my body's protective mechanism. What you do learn are coping strategies and how best to deal with what's happened. You never get over loss.

5- I Believe

As an avowed atheist I can say that I have had a renaissance, rather than a reincarnation. This is what the medical term post-morbid for somebody in my situation, would seem to imply. This seems a disturbing term, but although etymology is a real interest of mine, I fail to summon an equivalent.

The term post-morbid relating to something entirely different in doctors jargon is irrelevant, as the image of having died is something that it naturally conjures to a non-medic. Using what I deem to be inappropriate terms just because this derives from language set in stone, never seems productive, as specialised nomenclature is alienating rather than inclusive.

I'm sure that terms such as this continue to be used because we are so unaccustomed with having the medical-technology advanced enough to save somebody with a Brain Injury as severe as my own. For this reason I anticipate there being much more propaganda in the upcoming decades concerning Brain Injury. The numbers of people who can relate to somebody with a Brain Injury will surely dramatically increase. I think that obviously it is a good thing that so many more people with a Brain Injury will survive it being inflicted, only I would not having been through one, wish a Brain Injury on even my worst enemy. There is a fine line between those that should come round from a coma and those whom I think it would be tortuous to allow surviving. Difficulty resides in it being so difficult to gauge how much potential there is with each recovery. The quantity of time that you endure in a coma does not at all correlate with the state that you are in when you regain consciousness. Every Brain Injury is so unique, as is every brain.

The idea of existing amongst some fabricated paradise, detached from my friends and family doesn't appeal to the person that I know as myself. Religion's kudos seems to be principally based on the fact that I could never disprove it; by that measure I've slept with over one hundred outstandingly beautiful women. Yes I'll never have it proven that there cannot be some form of God / form of deities / re-incarnating force, though as I try to live my life fairly ethically, I don't really see that it can really be worth wasting my precious existence on preparing for death; in this respect I'm pretty much beyond even much caring.

We are confronted with enough controlling mechanisms in life without throwing religion into the mix. Using Daniel Defoe's sardonic example, that there is nothing more certain in life than death and paying taxes; thinking beyond that, religion seems to be obsolete. Not that I think that there is anything at all immoral or less intelligent with being at all religious; it is just the perpetrators of religions that can seem rather disturbed.

It is the finality of death that we seem so unable to cope with. Prior to 1988 it could be seen that I was dead. If looked at this way, things are less petrifying to understand. I find that dying's a great equaliser for us all.

Worse are clairvoyants. It is a bastion of our liberty to be able to believe in whatever we wish, though profiting from anybody's grief is amoral in my book. Taking advantage of bereaved people's weakness is beyond despicably manipulative. Of course I'm open to there being some sort of supernatural being; if you show me it I'll believe it.

Religious people I predict will claim how I lack the ability to think in abstract terms about our purpose. If this satisfies religious people, then they are more than welcome to think that. As things stand I'll continue to think that there is a 99.999 (recurring) per cent chance to me that there is no afterlife. When you're dead, then that's your lot. To me, religions just seem to complicate things in a life where we already have far too many tribulations. An inevitable outcome for us all is death, so wasting time devoting to the idea of an afterlife seems completely unnecessary.

Look at dietary requirements for religions if you are to argue that religion isn't a controlling mechanism. This obligation for people to justify things in the name of religion is rather depressing, considering how relatively brief our lives are. It seems rude not to take advantage of any opportunities of fun that we have. Perhaps there once was a useful place for religions in shaping societies morally; I'm fairly confident that one day, (in however many years it may take) religions will be anthropologically seen as archaic. There are magnitudes of things that can be exploited through religion. Perhaps this is why I find displayable forms of religion, most notably iconography, incredibly brash. It goes against human nature for it to be unfeasible to explain things, though creating something to have had trust in and unquestionably believing in it just doesn't credibly make any intelligent sense. A militant atheist is not a belief that I think I adhere. Verging on this is something that I cannot but help when it t is quite apparent that religion has been used towards or been misused to excuse many violent conflicts.

Sometimes believing in an afterlife of some form is something that I wish that I had the propensity for; but I can't, and won't pretend otherwise. My cynicism leads me to believe that loads of people do exactly this. Missing something is a thing that I often feel; given that such a vast quantity of people, far more intelligent than I am, believe in a religion. I'd do anything to be able to talk to loved ones again, so in this respect I really wish I was religious occasionally. If anything this only further confirms the fallacy of religion- fabricating something for convenience seems desperate, rather than informed.

Maybe it's a flaw in my character, but I can't believe in things because I just want to. As a child this was practised ('practise' perhaps being the wrong word as nothing about it has ever happened!) by me, though the knowledge of how silly this was is established by the fact that I'd be a rich and famous millionaire philanderer by the age that I am now. A sufficient replacement for religion seems to be faith in humanity and an interest in our wellbeing. The amount of greedy religious people undermines their beliefs so much in itself on its own. Without this and, good to people transnationally, I really fail to grasp what the point of religion now is.

A terrible element of religion and supernaturalism is that it can make perfectly sane people seem to be incredibly dependent on tales. Religions just seem to have a propensity to be always getting away with things based on avoidance of blame. What has come to annoy me is that sometimes at social gatherings religious people can be proud and go shoving it down your throats and go on about the beauty of their religious practise. This normally concerns an admirable quality, such as sharing and toleration. (Qualities that should exist anyway) Contrarily I find that if I was to go lauding it like that about my atheism, it would be considered fairly abrasive or just plain rude.

Frustration is an understated way of describing the confusion at why in the unwritten constitution of the UK; religious practise can still place a barrier towards our society's evolution. Civil partnerships are a prime example of demonstrating the redundancy of religion in shaping progress. The fact that we still need to give credit to religious opinion that differs from the overall consensus is nothing short of ridiculous. This explains why the majority of people that adhere to religion often must have to justify what they want believe using the label of faith.

Rationalism is something towards which I adhere. Religion is an antonym to rationality. From this perspective I can interpret that the cons of religion far outweigh the pros that they cause. They impose restraint rather than afford any freedom. It is depressing that people choose devotion to some higher sense of purpose, rather than attain enough fulfilment from the wonder of life. Opium of the masses was required in yesteryear when we were unable to attain a great deal beyond much fulfilment of life beyond sweat and toil. Now we have developed beyond this, so let's stop using belief as a way of keeping people down and just move on.

All that religion then does is offer a pathway for authorised bigotry. The vast majority of religious people are not bigoted, so now that we have finally arrived at an ethically based code of conduct, can't we all just reap the benefits of religion without naming the practise. As an irreligious person, it just seems rather redundant to practise something that lacks consistency in terms of the beliefs that society has provided you without religion existing. Without reiterating the point to excess, religion is not needed for progress to occur. Religion's frequently used by the people in power, for the people in power.

The brutal reality is that in many parts of the world I could be slaughtered for saying what I'm writing. I'm not being remotely aggressive. Well I'm not trying to tell you anything and prevent you from being free from believing whatever you like.

Culturally I understand how shying away from religion may be immensely difficult for some. Many of the cultural things that religions oversee are beneficial in themselves, though they could surely be done without believing in deities. Fasting, for example, seems like a fantastic way of learning to appreciate what we value and take for granted in life; though there needing to be some fable to back this up seems rather outdated in our technological age. Life's too short. My Granddad, all too accurately once said to me how, "as you get older, you really understand that like things, people never ever change." This explains why religion is one thing that has always persisted. What we all pretty much want is to be comfortable.

What religion can irrevocably place is a level of complication and pressure upon decision making that we really just don't need. It seems to place an extra dimension on decision making that people should be an awful lot freer without.

This is why, money, as much as it doesn't buy happiness, helps. Money as a conversation matter nauseates me fairly rapidly; unless you're genuinely starving, (and I don't mean saying that you are because you fancy a bite to eat...) there is never any real need to socially drop money in to the conversation. It's tasteless. My conclusion on the whole "living within your means" argument, is that frugality is fine, whereas stinginess and penny-pinching is not for people of reasonable wealth. I'm happy to do things such as buy other people drinks whilst I'm at the bar, as I'm just too lazy to waste more fun-time queuing and I'm not privileged enough to always financially justify this display of affluence.

As so often in my experience, many of the best ideas are heard within pubs. Recently during a 'philosophical' debate that was being had between me and a few others, a good friend (who studied biology at university) declared how there once was a need for religion to shape science. This goes along the lines of, (or so I interpreted anyway) you needing something to disprove in order to prove anything and this paved the development in knowledge. At the time, I'd drunk enough to think that this was genius. (I didn't admit this to him mind) After a good night's sleep, I still regard it as a pretty sound idea in terms of explaining science's relationship with religion.

Life throws many things at us that are difficult or impossible to grasp. Brain Injuries are notoriously complex to fully understand, despite millennia of study. Perhaps the calcification in my right elbow is perhaps a prime example of how we now prolong human life where my injury could not have been sustained in the past. Calcification involves the strange phenomenon of the body sprouting a new bone as it cannot comprehend the situation of prolonged unconsciousness. It was heterotypic-ossification in my case. As it was so eloquently related to me, my operation involved 'chiselling' the excess bone away from my right elbow. I'm pretty squeamish as it is, so good morphine's a relief. It is dangerous to say definitively how long ago I would not have been able to survive my injury. I just wouldn't feel comfortable hypothetically insinuating that I would have sustained my injury just ten years ago.

Feeling grateful for having experienced this surgery does not naturally sit all that well, as it was hardly something that was initially requested by me prior to being inflicted with the accident. Uncomfortable is something that has always been felt by me, at seeing any blood or guts being shown on any medical programme or violent scene. Eradicating this is something that has not fully being achieved yet. I can see how my queasiness with gore could be seen as a way of attention-seeking, in the same way that fussy-eaters can seem pathetic.

Maybe I'm just too much of a glutton to comprehend how somebody can ever object to food. What particular eaters could be in fact doing are just doing is just trying to exert some control, (there are children starving in this world etc. is my argument for why this is overly-indulgent) though you could easily shoot-me-down, claiming how treating injury is essential, though I can't really look at blood. Wastage is a thing that is never to anybody's benefit and this can extend to fussiness towards food, to trying to have a broad mind and trying to enjoy things in life. (However tenuous this link may be...) What we all must want is to be able to experience as many things in our brief lives as possible. Denying you alternative nutrition doesn't seem like a clever way of doing this.

Idealistically I'd just like for everybody to be happy and treat each other as fairly and equally as possible. My limited experience of religion refutes, rather than supports this thesis and I'm certainly never going to apologise for thinking this.

Religion seems to thrive off of making you feel that you need it. Life's a sufficient wonder for me in itself without needing to epitomise upon it through being servile to some fabricated theory.

It's depressing that many people around the world are unable to enjoy the beauty of this life without thinking that there must be something better. Through encouraging this belief, religion makes a mockery of the beauty afforded to us through this life.

6- Against All Odds

It can certainly be said that I have exceeded expectations. My parents were despicably informed at the Royal London when I was still in a coma, that I may never attain an independent life that great.

I would never have wanted to live without full command of my faculties, yet obviously I never had the onus of being able to choose. I really have been shown just how fragile everyone is and how it would be futile to devalue life, but by the same measure, life for life's sake isn't worth anything valuable in my view. I don't know why when medics cannot accurately foresee if I would survive functionally or not, they cannot be honest and just admit that they really have no idea how the situation will turn out, rather than only relate to relatives with a definition next to the ultimate worst.

On account of such distressing news being given to my bystanders, in collation with other things that I would categorise as disgraceful, I've come to find that indifference to it now is often the only way forward.

Despite the litigiousness of contemporary British society, I cannot comprehend honesty not always being the best policy. It would surely be ethically preferable for medics when they don't know, not to relate guises propagating some ill-informed (forgive the pun) opinion of how a situation will terminate. Pretending to be knowledgeable on something that you cannot be has the reverse effect of the trust that you're searching.

This opportunity shall be used by me to praise the Queen Elizabeth's Foundation (QEF) in Banstead, Surrey. I was there between September 2010 and June 2011. Ultimately, it serves the integral function of treating clients with their deserved dignity. It seems to recognise what an arduous process all clients are going through. The most exceptional thing about rehabilitation units is that none of their clients are ever ending up there through initial choice. Of course, this is not to say that

I never witnessed a client being spoken to in a slightly derogatory manner at the QEF, though this was infinitely seldom. Perhaps I am the one misinterpreting the occasional instance of a client being mistreated through being overly defensive of Brain Injury victims.

One thing that I do not suffer gladly is fools, especially ones who have got no real excuse to be that way. Wherever you reside there always seem to exist a significant proportion of dense people and one of the most testing things about being disabled is finding your judgement automatically sacrificed to professionals. Vexing (without being too eighteenth-century period drama) is how I can now describe the feeling of being seen as beneath adults who are certainly not always the sharpest knife in the drawer.

The vast preponderance of therapists at the QEF were fantastic people and comfortable is not something that I'd feel for any of the staff there to feel like my slating is at-all directed at them. The phenomenal work they did for me is really appreciated highly and real admiration is something that I have for nearly all of the workers at the QEF. They do a far superior job than I ever would at their vocation; patience is something that is not had in a great quantity by me and this is essential to be a therapist. The QEF managed to rescue me from detachment that I could so easily feel in at planning revolving around me, that I could feel I had absolutely no influence over initially.

As I've tried to make apparent, the complexity of how precisely the brain functions is exemplified by the fact that we still have both atheism and religion at opposite ends of the strata. Agnosticism can be seen to cover-up the middle ground, though surely once you've come to accept that there will never be any solid proof, you must go into either the believer or non-believer camp. Some people just appear to be craving the confidence to express what they really think; it is no easy task, given how fierce religions can be. Finding alternative ways of explaining circumstances that deviate from whatever you prescribed religion's norms are cannot be easy.

I was lucky enough to have always been able to grasp the full extent of my injury, although the learning of many things is a gradual process. The term 'insight' is popular for professionals to throw around for this. Sometimes this appears to be misconstrued; nobody in humanity can surely know how they'll do in all aspects of life before things actually happen. What was confirmed to me relatively quickly after I became conscious from my coma circa April 2010 was just how much of a difficulty my situation was to all that knew me. I use the approximate term circa, as coming around from a coma really is a gradual process. I wasn't fully aware of how inadvertently privileged I was in so many respects. Without intending to sound flippant, I have gone beyond all initial predictions of how feasibly I would be able to recover.

It cannot be helped but being made to feel tiresome by me that I was obliged to justify even the most seemingly trivial transaction that I undertook. I do recognise the awkward position that people in my situation must put therapists in, as they are not liable to automatically know one iota about me. An overly structured lifestyle is something that is found difficult. Like it or not, a success in life seems to normally depend on some routine, though choice over where to go in life is something we are all reliant upon. In this respect, part of therapeutic success has involved jumping through hoops. Such as removing myself from the Court of Protection (that I was automatically placed under, whilst out of consciousness) is an ultimate example of this contradiction in terms; like me supposedly receiving protection, though having to initially get permission to use my own money!

The idea of having a court of protection is an oxymoronic concept worth rivalling Christian Science.

I'm left with principally my tangible deficits to recover from. I still suffer from ataxia. This is a neurological sign of a gross lack of muscle co-ordination as a result of damage to the cerebellum which affects my nervous system. This has really changed the sound of my voice. I'm just glad that I was never an opera singer, as this confusion with the way in which my muscles are communicated with by being sent impulses from my brain. It even made the most mundane task of transporting a mug of tea from my kitchen to my living room hard work. Developing more advanced compensatory strategies with dealing with ataxia has been the way forward.

Ataxia can wane, though I think that I will always suffer from some traces of it. My specific ataxia has now been defined by physiotherapists as weak. Much of my ataxia was labelled in me when in reality much of my ataxic symptoms resided in apparent neurological muscle weakness. This exemplifies just how complex it is categorising the results of a Brain Injury.

What I've really been able to appreciate in such a foreseeable way is just how interconnected all aspects of rehabilitation are. For example as my physical core-stability and dexterity improves, my ataxia can show signs of declining and my voice dramatically improves. Now, whilst I recognise that the sound of my voice may not be exactly what it was before, I am able to speak clearly. I definitely can understand why Pride is one of the Seven Deadly Sins. What has been an ultimate test for me is not to automatically assume that my altered voice makes me sound inferior. More luck can be extracted from the fact that I am a heterosexual male as women at least appear to be far 'deeper' when it comes to choosing a partner.

Self-obsessed is something of an understatement for the way that I was as I was in the process of witnessing constant inspection of my life.

Being audacious I could claim that at least I had an excuse to be this way. I'm sure that we all have friends or at least acquaintances that could only be described as self-absorbed.

One of the things post formal recovery that I have learned is that it's incredibly infantile and unappealing to always be talking about your own business. Growing-up should make you learn that nobody really cares that much about your every concern.

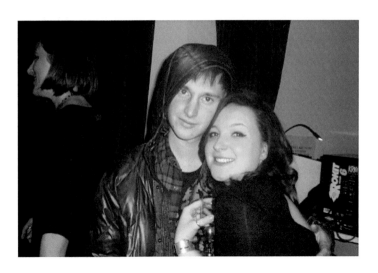

Jack and Carrie

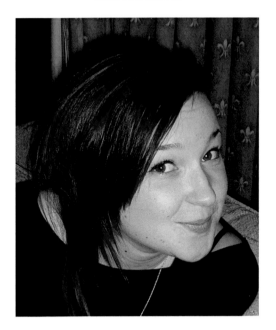

Carrie

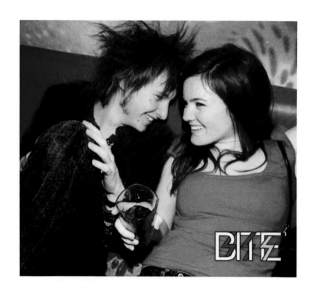

Jack and Chelsea

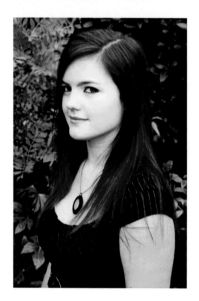

Chelsea

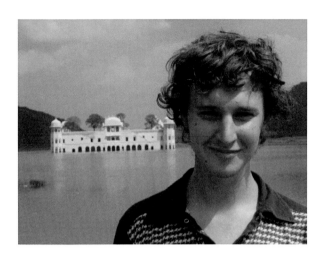

Jack

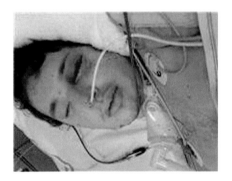

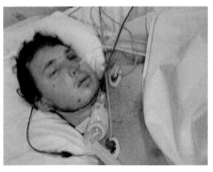

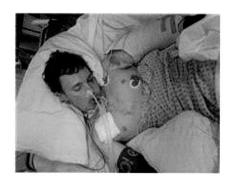

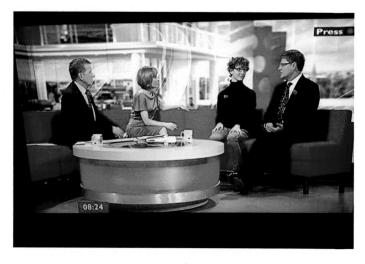

On BBC News, 3rd November, 2011

7- Rock Bottom

Initially in June 2010 I was unequivocally informed that my memory functions had been severely impaired. A particularly scary element of Brain Damage regards the fact that the part of the brain that has been damaged can never be repaired. What is gone is gone.

As I'm still only young my brain is still pliable, so that upon having a TBI my brain can just learn new ways of functioning to compensate for what has been lost. I still object to people who do not know a thing about me from Adam, having the audacity to coldly relate such sensitive information amidst lots of disconnected professionals in a room. I would have assumed that medical staff should have a more sophisticated grasp of ethics that to put a patient through such overt subjugation.

There has long being ground-breaking propaganda concerning the mistreatment of patients and the deplorable consequences of mistreating the ill. There is something immensely utilitarian, rightly or wrongly about the ways of interpreting and relating data in the medical profession. Assessments are indispensable guidelines, but they're not to be concretely trusted, overriding everything else.

One of the most invaluable lessons for me has been learning to trust my own judgement again. This is hard when you have been told that due to damage to your temporal lobe, you can have severe trouble memorising information. As stated, initially I was related the memory deficits that I had somewhat callously and condescendingly. I can only really summon the adjective of depraved in the organisation of this process. This is on account of the bulk of my problems being related to a rather large audience without my presence, let alone permission.

It is still felt by me that being related information by professionals is rather like being branded with cast-iron. The memory problems that I had have recovered substantially since then. The QEF psychologists observed that the forefront of my problem lay with recalling, rather than retaining information. Upon an assessment on my prospective memory (allowing for prompts to be used), it was found to be 'average'. Never has the word 'average' given me so much elation. What is essential is acceptance and confidence of the way in which life changes. You cannot have one of those things without the other. It resonates in confronting what elements have altered since your injury; outright denial of anything is never beneficial. It tends to rank alongside forwardness in terms of trying to delude yourself by not confronting reality.

There was a lot of necessity in conducting memory assessments on me. Only I do feel that this information could have been communicated to me in a more empathetic way and related to me in an open rather than clandestine manner.

I can't dispute the findings of memory assessments, only I feel that there would be a lot to be gained if doctors were not so perpetually dogmatic with qualitative evidence. The memory assessments that were conducted on me were integral to my recovery, yet are tainted with elements of futility as there can never be an accurate comparison with my PRE-MORBID memory. I now use a similar technique homosexuality has used with the word 'queer' with post-morbid; I can use it although I am still adverse to others taking the liberty. I oppose the use of any terminology that only provides such an inept categorisation of a situation.

Obviously no man is an island and I have always vehemently believed this; independence is something which I have always strove for. Sounding like a right impetuous little wretch, I've always objected to being told what to do by anybody. (Ask my close childhood relatives on that) Using animalistic imagery, I felt like a guinea-pig throughout formalised therapy. Sadly I am part of the tested generation.

Sometimes it appeared offensive for it to be assumed that you may be unaware that you are under covert examination. Empirical qualitative data on my memory functions is valid, yet also incredibly reliant on aspersions. I comprehend doctors' vehement trust in assessment criteria, there should just be more recognition of how individualised their assessment results are. I can vouch for the fact that being disparagingly told that my memory was flawed will eternally be imprinted on my brain. Ultimately I could just have never envisaged a situation so bleak ever occurring throughout my entire life.

Without prompts being used in assessment around June 2011 my memory unaided came up as 'low-average' on an assessment. Like the vast majority of tests conducted on me, I have absolutely zilch idea of where my memory would have fallen prior to my accident occurring. Presumably it would have been better then. Now I have no conception of where my memory would fall on any such tests, though as it serves all of my required functions in life I'm pretty much beyond even much caring.

Integral to identity is a conception of self. Thankfully my conception of self never remotely altered, though it is a card that is difficult to juggle against being interrogated persistently. Having a Brain Injury affords many with the presumption that you must be different.

This is scary. As any receiver of discrimination shall be aware, it is both petrifying and infuriating should not even begin to capture what it feels like to be defined through something completely beyond your control. Categorising things in through blanket terms goes beyond exposing ignorance to go as far as being a clear display of insecurity in that you want to solidify some unity with "your kind". What I've found traumatising is this belief that due to the wounding of my brain there must be something lost within my thought process. Yes, there have clearly been some subtle alterations to my cognition, but not remotely to my character.

When you are significantly handicapped the line between physicality and cognition in people's eyes get blurred. This helps to ensure that the line of normality gets blurred in any patient's eyes.

8- Poker Face

Idiosyncrasies are sometimes what you most miss being institutionalised. Cringeworthy as you may occasionally confess to finding them, without so being you find your identity significantly encroached. Everything in my life had always tried to be enacted in a casual approach. This is an element of your lifestyle that it is hard to retain upon being inflicted by something as intense as a Brain Injury. I always found assumptions deeming that I was not fully aware of my situation cruel. You certainly compartmentalise different traits of your personality and I can certainly say that I know myself as impeccably as I ever want to, especially succeeding a Brain Injury.

Being surrounded by people that you can trust has always being integrally important to me; as I'm no misanthrope it has always been doable. Without having this I just feel lonely and there can never be anything healthy in isolation. Learning to properly appreciate my own company again has been a worthy lesson.

Without deliberately glamorising the past I feel that as much I would have deplored the label conformist as an adolescent, this is probably what I ticked the boxes to be. I recognise that going along a conventional route often appears to be different things for everybody. Principally I've always strove for a fun and easy life. I've come to believe that frequently rule breakers must be insecure themselves, as by disobeying any authority, you're automatically reliant on others doing the same. You must naturally feel venerable being forced to reside on the outskirts of society; I've come to have some faith in the idea of their being a branch best described as an underclass. Not in the traditional sense of the word, but certainly in that there appear a growing number of people feeling completely alienated from society's procedures.

Generalisations have the intrinsic flaw of always overlooking individuality. Individuality is difficult to propagate when you feel so propagated. I have always had the reputation amongst many friends and family members of being like an elephant with certain aspects of my memory, yet potentially being scatter-brained in others. The bulk of this now, as then, broadly appears to relate to what you're interested in. Although I can only vouch for myself, I would presume that this is universal. What I have found has been incredibly beneficial to me is a basic understanding of the ways in which the memory functions. I'm convinced that your memory must be engineered towards your own particular interests.

A self-fulfilling prophecy about my future prospects based on my accident is something that I'm desperately trying to avoid. This is what I believe what would have happened if I had given too much authority to professionals that are not known by me (i.e. strangers') opinion. What is difficult is being forced to have to carve out your own identity again at the age of 21 whilst you feel that you get treated like a child. Constantly being given the opinion that your maturity is being questioned is incredibly condescending.

The format of supposed lessons in rehabilitation felt at times like something of a mockery. To use an example, I always felt that I had quite a broad knowledge of disciplines such as Personal, Social and Health Education. (PSHE) Underestimated is something that was frequently felt by me and this can transcended into an undermined sense of self-worth.

It often felt that the concept of you in fact having a fair amount of knowledge on a given area can be unintentionally overlooked within rehabilitation and this feels especially demeaning. It was found immensely difficult to have to tolerate being automatically grouped with similar people on account of having suffered a TBI. The ordeal of enduring a Brain Injury is undeniably something that we all experienced, though that is certainly not a fundamental personality trait in itself. This felt at times like you were relied upon to tolerate being treated as though you did not possess the authority to question circumstances.

It being presumed that you are not equipped with the ability to interpret information feasibly was immensely difficult for me to tolerate. Rightly or wrongly, intelligence was always something upon which considerable value was placed in my mind. Having this element of your persona under constant questioning was something soul-destroying. I'll admit that I can be overly sensitive and this does not help matters. Going with proverbs, being told some things felt rather like teaching your granny to suck eggs. Luckily the old repetitive nod is something that I've long been equipped with thanks to principally my mother; you can satisfy people by letting them know that you're listening, whilst secretly totally ignoring many things that they say. Listening and taking notice of other people's advice is usually invaluable, though it's found better by me, to be selective over which pieces of advice you take account of rather than automatically taking what anybody says as gospel.

A stage of no longer feeling the necessity to compare every aspect of my life to how it was before the accident, has been reached. The best thing now is that it has been a considerable time since I departed formalised rehabilitation and this means that I can justify my actions in the same way as anybody else. The disparaging nature in my character shows itself here, as a TBI sufferer things can seemingly be exploited to make things easier for professionals if they presume that you have inferior astuteness, as you are disabled.

Sometimes the thing found most frustrating, was the fact that I was being treated in a way that is dismissive of your PRE-MORBID credential. An element that was found to be difficult by me was that you could be grouped with people with a Brain Injury and it to be assumed that you were all of the same calibre. This of course is not to say that others had automatically any lower abilities than me in any way; we were just different.

Comedy is the only way at which I am able to now view many of the situations that I found myself confronted with.

This is not a criticism of anybody, but more a reflection of the generalised circumstances that I found myself cooped-up within. A black sitcom reliant on dark-humour seems like my only answer to dealing with this. Attempting to make a wry or tongue-in-cheek comment about appropriate things had always constituted the bulk of my conversation. It is a challenging trait to pull-off when you find yourself being viewed as a 'patient' with significantly altered speech.

Your capacities are fervently being questioned under rehabilitation and your reliability is disregarded. This was particularly difficult for both me and therapists as my voice was hardly speaking in a way easy to interpret what I had said. Psychologically it always felt that you would automatically perform less well at whatever task you were given to complete as I felt that the sound of my voice made me sound inferior.

Part of the problem probably lies in the fact that I was fairly shallow. This comes in terms of attaching unfounded amounts of value to the way in which you are defined, through there being some supposed basis of "normality" through which everybody is judged. Whilst the label of being "regular" or "standard" is something that I'd never have been remotely attracted to, conventional would certainly be rather accurate way to define the aspirations that I had in life.

In terms of playing towards strengths, it can be maintained by me, that I can have a rather phenomenal episodic memory. Close friends of mine are still at a loss as to quite how I am able to share countless anecdotes from our primary school days- even occurrences that we would rather forget. Many periods of my life seem to be encoded well in my brain due to my sociability and need to sequence the order in which things happen to fully understand how people relate to one another. There can be no decent gossip without doing that; it's supposedly been found that men do in fact spread gossip more than women, so I'll give no further defence.

This love of information about people has allowed me to retain a fantastic memory for dates. I seem to effortlessly be able to encode verbal memories to my brain. Visual episodes are a different matter. My visual memory, as I believe it, has always been comparatively abysmal. I think that part of the beauty of being an adult is having the proficiency to be rather coy about whatever deficits you believe your memory to have. My photographic memory always made action films, where there were numerous characters in the same costume often hard for me to follow. Avoiding action films seemed to me a rather obvious remedy.

Prior to having a Brain Injury it was never my responsibility to advertise my potential deficits. This is sure to be met with vehement disagreement from many Bachelor of Arts (BA) studiers, but I can conclude that my value in the power of words, over that of action makes me the archetypal literary student. (Apologies as I know that I'm stupidly sounding all pretentiously lah-di-da here)

There is luck to be extracted from the fact that I am a fuelled person, so that being told that I had a damaged memory, provided the requisite zest to build my memory functions to disprove assumptions that I grossly lacked the ability to retain information. This is not just me being defensive, as my memory was indeed badly damaged, yet I always think that ways of relating information are essential. I would strongly recommend 'The Man Who Mistook his Wife for a Hat' by Oliver Sacks to anybody wishing to gain some understanding of Brain Damage and just how reliant you are on our memory we all are. I find the way that the memory works fascinating; it is crucial to the way you understand anything. As mentioned in the Oliver Sacks book, your memory works so subconsciously in how you can regurgitate information.

A poignant example came over a take-away curry, when suddenly I was able to spontaneously recount my Dad saying "Jack, Jack it is Dad" at the time when I was very slowly coming out of my coma. It is remarkable how your brain encodes pieces of information. It is odd that I can recall this snippet so accurately, though until an instant before I seemingly had no recollection of it whatsoever.

From my experiences of apparent memory loss, I advise that you always try to work around things to resolve them before you automatically accept them as your and other people's fortune. Never just assume that you can say whatever you like to a person because they will not be able to remember things.

9- Once in a Lifetime

Life will never be how I originally envisaged it to be throughout my twenties. This accident has ensured that my entire time will always have alternative goals and appreciation than what I planned.

It is something that I find incredibly disconcerting to think of the amount that was undertaken upon my body without my awareness.

This goes beyond my ever fading tracheotomy scar and clear scars on both of my upper arms. Things such as my processing speed and coping-strategies with dealing with the quadrant of blindness in my left eye I can also work to adjust to as best as possible. Things such as proficiency of your memory and processing-speed are terribly difficult to equate, as life never otherwise presents a standardised assessment of your pre-morbid credentials in such things. Whatever lasting damage shows up in assessment, more internally my psychological scars shall never be eradicated.

I don't think that I ever want them to, as recognising 'I' without them would be no easy task anymore. I shall also never recover from two of my loves dying. As with ninety-nine percent of the population I was never fully appreciative of my life. I am striving not to sound simplistic enough to think that we can ever live life in an accurately hierarchical way. A trip to developing country such as Asia or Africa (places that I'm hugely appreciative that I've been able to visit) is something that I would advocate to really try to understand more about the human psyche. Having independently travelled there before my accident, I consider that maybe I am relatively well placed to comment. I maintain that getting arrested in Malawi (it felt very Brigit Jones) as I ignorantly traversed its border with Tanzania without getting my passport stamped, remains the most petrified I have ever been. What travel has really made clear to me is just the quantity of things that we take for granted. Rather bourgeois is something that I unfortunately feel I sound here!

This attitude of being rather unappreciative of the quantity of luxuries that we have is becoming increasingly prevalent throughout Britain. Clearly there is no real exception in me. Whatever may be claimed we are clearly an awful distance from a true meritocracy and overall equality can sadly never be reached within the imminent future. To sound like an old codger, (maybe I was born in the wrong decade) but generations are all becoming increasingly spoilt and unaware of the intense labour involved in producing their goods.

Socialism now seems like a phenomenon that will have to be global rather than just internal. The exploitation amongst the West seems like it shall inevitably backfire; to be incredibly self-interested, I hope that this is after my lifetime. The accident has certainly acted to illustrate to just what a degree I could be blasé about what was allowed by my chosen lifestyle.

Idealism without any realism in claiming to be anti-Western often just makes people appear like complete hypocrites. Incongruously it is often the most privileged individuals that can claim to be the most dissatisfied with the way developed countries are governed. These individuals are ardently too happy to capitalise on the advantages afforded to us. The insincerity of these individuals is all too apparent.

Children who are too spoilt will inexorably lose out in the long-race of life, when they're forced to learn that life just doesn't work quite like that! In reality the mort protective that you can seem to be of children (and I'm certainly not yet a parent) is to let them learn from taking their own risks. What happened to me really highlights how you can't afford to be over-protective of any loved ones, as much as you may have the natural urge to do exactly that. What is somewhat scary is to what quantity everything is disposable in wealthier countries this increasingly consumer age.

What is increasingly alarming is the disparity in the evolution of countries across the world. The rapid advancement in technology has revolutionised the entire globe.

Attitudes towards many things have completely changed. Without the nineties Labour government's Freedom of Information Act, news is now just far more accessible to everybody than it ever at all was in the past. There is another paradox in the fact that things being unendingly available are a fantastic thing, though it has significantly changed our attitude towards many of society's social constructions.

Take going on holidays for example; whilst it was once considered an essential time to completely detach you and relax, this is now impossible. Things such as laptops, kindles and iPhones mean that communication is always accessible and our brains can always be made busy. It's changing education dramatically, as there is no longer any real need to recite things, as you can effortlessly find out within seconds.

Abstract reasoning now seems key to making any worthy input to a vast array of different activities. Connectable is something that you always are within modernity, it has completely changed our organisational habits and general time-keeping. Back-up meeting agendas and having to rely on your sense of direction and geographical knowledge are now redundant.

Much of our approach to thinking about things has been completely eroded. To further confirm to me, in existence of another world, there is the fact that compared to just a couple of generations ago, magic has already been achieved. I'm sure that my ancestors would have thought you stark raving mad if you communicated to them an idea of having a wide array of information connecting the globe at your fingertips. The irony that this has brought is forcing you to plan relaxation and deliberately disconnect yourself at times for ease. Embracing this rather than shy-away from it is the only real way without undoing technological progress. The rapidity at which the world moves was confirmed to me recently on a television documentary, stating how portable chip and pin payment machines were only established in 2004! The paces at which things can be taken for granted is staggering and go yet further to confirm our adaptability.

10- Set Me Free

The crux of any reassurance throughout my engagement in the therapeutic process has been that my spiritual identity (detached from any supernatural connotations) has remained untarnished throughout my experience. This is why it has struck me as so unnerving, being shown data confirming that elements of my cognitive functioning have dramatically altered post-TBI. Being confronted with any information about yourself that you have no conception of is distressing. The accident has certainly made me accustomed with just how vulnerably fragile we all are. Any delusional notion of invincibility that I may have had has undoubtedly been quashed.

Changes include a reduced processing speed, which now falls within the low end of the average spectrum. I can only presume that it would have been higher before. Difficulty resides in there being absolutely no official record of my processing speed prior to having a Brain Injury. I can understand why processing speed may have reduced as due to my brain being so colossally damaged, I've had to resurrect new pathways to constitute processing pieces of information.

Things have had the potential of being especially hard for me to deal with as the accident has starkly exposed to me just how much I could take falling alongside society's supposed academic elite for granted. The term elitism is deplorable in itself. There is now a stark line between me now viewing the Brain Injury that I've suffered as being a definitive episode of my life rather than something through which I'm defined. It now feels as though I've reclaimed the ability to hold as much faith in my own opinion. What has never been accepted by me is the thought of ending up with an inferior quality of life to that which I would have had prior to the accident occurring. At the age of twenty-one, adulthood had never properly begun being lived, so it is hard to base my overall monetary compensation. Quantifying the intangible is what my recovery is based upon.

The difficulties with my processing speed are mainly what spoil my memory. There is absolutely no problem with me encoding and retaining information, though due largely to my reduced processing speed, retracting it may take longer than before. In my speech I suffer from mild dysarthria, which is a motor speech disorder resulting from a neurological injury.

No longer do I suffer from any aphasia; more from what we all suffer (not being able to find the precise word you're looking for). To me it has become apparent that word summoning difficulty usually lies in the inability to be anything close to the definition of your lost word. I've found that once you begin to attempt to contextualise the word you are searching for, it reappears with rapidity. Synonyms are no potential remedy for aphasia, as without an accurate situation at which to use the word, any attempts at finding it are redundant. I do not feel that I'm being self-protective when I say that I think that the frustration of temporary word loss is something to which we can all relate. I used to experience it to the extreme, now I do not feel I encounter it at much beyond the average level. This exemplifies the fact that once many neurological deficits are found they are often widely found, only like many other things exaggerated in your case.

It is imperative to be aware of the fact that nobody is ever devoid of making stupid mistakes. I think that this is sometimes what therapists can overlook when talking to you. For me, the transition from having led a largely independent life into a controlled institution was perhaps the hardest thing to take. As stated, I have the flaw here of occasionally being overly proud. I have never had a politically neo-liberal agenda, so consequentially appreciate that no man can ever be totally independent.

Cynicism is not something that I believe is clever in any way and trying to get laughs out of cynicism is not something that I'd ever be proud of. Only perhaps confirmation that I can by nature be rather cynical in that I believe that doubt and honesty are often not that far separated.

Whilst admiration for people in the caring profession is something that I have, making mountains out of molehills is something that I frequently feel is performed in order to validate their constant requirement.

Understanding that we are all heavily reliant on each other for any progress was part of growing-up for me. I hope that it doesn't sound contradictory for me to declare that I have always been highly adverse to patronisation. It must be appreciated though, that patronisation has to be accepted as an integral role that is crucial to many worthy therapy jobs.

Although I have departed officialised rehabilitation, I still consider myself in a therapeutic circumstance; part of me thinks that as life is ever a learning curve for us all. Certainly, adjusting to many different things, is something I have had to do. Regurgitating specific information is harder than it used to be I think. Lacking an accurate comparison with your abilities PRE-MORBIDLY is frustrating. Occasionally I got the impression that people felt that they were being shrewder in being able to observe some changes in any of my characteristics.

As mentioned, there were many observations were made about my behaviour and I'll maintain that many alterations were purely circumstantial. Sinking to a rather base level of retaliation now, but try being incapacitated involuntarily and see how well you respond before you nonchalantly throw about comments.

Going on with my cynicism, it just seems that some therapists are far too overly reliant on being able to 'assist' you with all things to justify their job. Of course the jobs that they serve are invaluable and a lot of respect for therapists is needed, only at times they fail to recognise quite how condescending some of their requests feel. It can feel rather excruciating. To the same degree as I object to being patronised, therapists understandably loath by being seemingly outsmarted by TBI sufferers. At times comparisons can be drawn between it seeming at times to simplify therapists if you are ignorant. This is where honesty seems like a better way than cynicism in describing the discomfort at describing how it feels being constantly instructed. No matter to what extent your best interests are at heart, every single footstep of your chosen life-path feeling like it is under some obligation to be externally analysed feels incredibly diminishing.

Some things are clearly more equitable than others. Vision is a one area that I feel was neglected in my rehabilitation. This isn't a criticism as I have had to be forced to know that optometry is incredibly complex and my eyesight was not an initial priority. Reassured, rather than disappointed is what I would describe my feelings upon it being confirmed that I did indeed have a noticeable defect in the form of my eyes lacking fusion. In turn this means that there is a problem with their convergence of the left eye. In layman's terms, I'll describe this as having a lazy eye; what is damaged as my eye's ability to fully collate what it sees. This does not at all show up on standard optical tests. Coping strategies again come into play; especially essential here as, (presumably like any BA degree) I always have lots of reading to be persevering with.

The complication in defining my precise visual deficiencies is further evidence of the complexity of neurology. Another possible assistance that I could have for my eyes (which I couldn't help but suppress a snigger upon being mentioned) is Botox injections. As I just about understood it, (and I have extremely limited optical knowledge) this would have the effect of paralysing my left eye, so that the eyes would be forced to subconsciously relearn to converge gradually. As vain as I may or may not have been, I certainly would never consider having any Botox at the 'tender' age of twenty-one.

I cannot help but be capable of conducting myself far more stoically than ever before. Perhaps I am just being rather too offhand in saying this; it is only really when a tragedy like mine occurs that you can ever know how you will deal with it.

It never feels like I am devoid of empathy in any way, or fail to see things from other people's perspective and have undoubtedly proved myself to be more resilient than ever anticipated since my Brain Injury. Relishing the fact that I can still get worried about relatively mediocre things is something that has assured me. This is the sort of guarantee that I am the same as ever that I needed. The fact that I can prioritise things much more accurately than ever before, hardly justifies being brain injured to me. Being degraded in having to relearn the most fundamental characteristics is a natural consequence of being attached to a feeding tube and catheter, which is no pleasant experience, but necessary. One of the only benefits that I feel I have learned from this is the inclination that I can more accurately prioritise what I do with life.

This is why it has been so vital for me to reclaim control. Every element of my autonomy was removed from my person; it is starkly obvious which people have a conception of this and those that are totally unmindful of this. Having to 'de-robe' (without being overly regal) and then paraded stark-naked in a shower whilst somebody of the opposite sex 'supervised' you wash was hardly agreeable. It ties-in with the entire feeling of losing any desirability under all circumstances.

You feel like your liberty has been sacrificed throughout hospitalisation, without being surrendered. Although I'd never consider myself to be a prude or exhibitionist, this is still uncomfortable. At the age of am, appearing naked in front of a female would normally have a sexual, rather than a hygienic motive.

Finding independence diminished, feels incredibly demeaning, as the entire circumstance of residing in a hospital is just horrific. It is the idea of being requested to do things that you never foresaw yourself having to do that is barely durable. Tempting-fate is a thing that I obviously do not wish to do, although being embarrassed does not come as easily to me as it once would have done. Society in general just appears to always be opening-up and as a whole, becoming far less inhibited. In my generation for example, being embarrassed to talk about sex amongst friends and swearing is far more the exception than the norms. Conversely old-fashioned phenomena such as racial or sexist slurs have become incredibly unacceptable. Rightly so too, though they are far from eradicated in a covert way; homophobia and general bigotry unfortunately persist. Broadly speaking they reside as the omission rather than the norm. As society now appears so individualised, it is just no longer possible to make the same generalisations and defining yourself separately seems to be our optimum goal.

As much as stupidly attempting to be something of a hipster (even though I'd deplore the label and categorisation) had become part of my identity, a job, house, wife and 2.4 children would easily have featured on my life-path. If allergic to the damn creatures is something that I was a dog is something that I'd easily own – being shown the hard way that allergies were not an attention seeking device is no fun! Like other people can be, I'd always been fairly dismissive of allergies. Now I'm trying to learn that you cannot afford to be dismissive of anything. In an unfathomable way, understanding the hardships inflicted on people by things that other people take for granted is a microcosm of society's inequalities. As much as hating the label is something that I would always have done, it is fair to say that my agenda for living life as a whole was pretty predictable and this seemed practical.

11- Deeper Feelings

The Royal London nurses still call me their 'little miracle', which when accompanied by flattery and compliments from my friends and relatives really helps to ensure that I get better. I am just privileged to have the heartfelt support of so many inspirational people. This is what fuels me to persevere with my recovery.

Telling me that I can no longer do something could not give me more ammunition to recover in getting better; assumptions deeming you less capable than you wish to be are incredibly rewarding to disprove. Certainly having had no say in the matter of the accident happening on the 1st of January 2010 is something to deal with, but I can orchestrate certain elements of my recovery. I am clearly no deity, so I can be sure that it is only down to luck and determination that have allowed me to recover thus far.

Part of me is simply resolute to always reassure myself of how positive my attitude towards life is. After having spent an entire year avoiding being on the brink of tears, I'll hopefully never return to that destitute state again.

There were elements of the cognitive difficulties that I faced made familiar to my maternal family by my Nan, who had suffered the immortalising Alzheimer's disease. With bitter-irony I'd had several conversations expressing how a mental impairment is ultimately the scariest thing that I'd ever want to suffer from. The fundamental difference between a TBI and Alzheimer's involves the pattern of recovery. This is where Alzheimer's could be called an antonym to a TBI, in terms of Alzheimer's being purely degenerative.

What is particularly distressing with the condition of Alzheimer's is that it seems to entirely dismiss a person's previous credential in the eyes of observers. A dream is something that I interpret that Alzheimer's feels like to the sufferer. The hard thing about both conditions is that relatives can be forced with having to witness seeing their loved ones existing only in a bodily form. This is tortuous on both accounts. It is difficult to be faced with people that you have always speculated as having emerged quite victorious from the gene-pool, being so fundamentally reduced.

In many ways, as pointed out in a book written by Nicholas Fearn on philosophy, handicaps such as Alzheimer's confirm the fallacy of religion to me. If you lose every aspect of your being whilst you're still alive, then what chance is there, you're officially dead? I predict the calls claiming that the purpose and essential meaning of religion is being completely lost by me. Perhaps so, but whilst my life continues to pass whilst I clearly have a lack of any soul, my logic forces me to utterly dismiss religion.

Occasionally jealousy is something that is had by me towards religious people as it must provide some comfort. Though at least I don't have to put on any sort of pretence, which I'm convinced that is exactly what many religious people are doing. The sociologist Steve Bruce once stated that religion will be dead within thirty years, (and that was in the nineties, so it seems an impossibility now!) though at times of great austerity, the comfort-blanket of religion seems precisely what people want to turn to. Religious solace seems to me something that we go looking for rather than vice versa.

It can be frustrating to observe how people can be so consumed with their own life and ignorant judgements to really identify with sufferers of a cognitive impairment. From experience, psychological impairments can be extremely challenging to fully understand in adolescence, but adults should be able to truly empathise more. People in their formative years are always capable of understanding some things greater than any adult.

Excusing your children always, because they're too young to understand often seems unnecessary. People have the capacity to always make changes, but a nasty child is nearly always continuously a nasty adult. What people always seem to be in want of is taking responsibility for various actions. I'm incredibly grateful that my parents always treated me the same as anybody else; it seems most constructive to just treat people however they may act. Most children are always capable of responding if they want to; by this measure, you shouldn't need to give-in to them. Perhaps this is all far too easy for me to say, as I'm not with any offspring. Mollycoddled kids are often just too annoying as they can seem like just spoilt brats. To me, the most essential element of growing-up is adjusting to accommodate you in the world and learning to be happy throughout life. Some independence is essential, as you can only learn by making your own mistakes and picking-up the pieces seems essential. Being over-protected, you just never seem so accomplished at rectifying mistakes. Learning that we all make a significant amount of mistakes seems paramount. If you're not given permission to be away from the leach, fending for yourself adequately does not seem likely.

12- I've got to admit it's getting better

On both sides of my extended family, the knock-on effects of my accident can be acutely felt. On my dad's side for example, my grandparent's 60th Wedding Anniversary was spoilt by the fact that there could not be the given collaborative celebration given that I was unconsciously hospitalised. It cannot be overstated just how much the secondary effects of the accident that I was in have been overlooked. There shall always be many birthdays and Christmases without all of the loved ones that you would have spent time with being present. Rather than feeling only grief, I have now reached a stage at which I can just celebrate how privileged I have been to have known certain people.

As of now I have already reached the stage of acceptance to attain a more than adequate level of existence. I can now confidently refute assumptions that I have a greatly reduced mental capacity. I think that I am the only one who can really draw a valid comparison with me prior to my injury. In truth I'm beyond caring what other people record of such matter as I know that my intellectual ability can be used as it was before. The ordeal of a Brain Injury will remain eternally etched on my brain, though it is a chapter of my life which I can now close. Life will not necessarily transpire to be better or worse than prior to my injury; just different. Getting unleashed for the second time in life was a laboriously testing process, but it was always the ultimate aim of mine. In this respect I can be grateful for having the flexibility of never being philosophically conservative. Initially succeeding my accident I was scared of what my future held. This fear has elapsed as I now have no less excitement or tentative nerves than the average twenty-three year old. Anticipation is the gusto of life and questionably the most taxing thing I found about 2010 was that I never had anything of any significance to look forward to. If I did, it had always been arranged by another person, rather than coming naturally off my own back in a busy life. Now I find it quite liberating that several people (and I have managed to have kept this to an incredibly slight number) have now seen me at my most-intense state of grief. In many ways I am even more comfortable with these people than I could ever have been with anyone and I have real admiration for how they conducted themselves visiting me in hospital.

Another thing that I have had to reclaim is trust for everybody in my own abilities. There is a fine line between appreciating everything about you as exactly the same as prior to the injury and those who appear too absorbed in their own largely irrelevant misdemeanours, to know a real thing about you. This may sound self-absorbed, but it seems to be the most simplistic way of expressing divisions between people since my injury. My opinion in general of the human race has thankfully raised, yet I know who my friends are and who shall never be a true friend of mine; I'll still try to be perfectly amicable with everyone. Yet I know that those with whom my opinion has significantly deteriorated will never be mutual friends anymore. People that have failed to offer me invaluable support are fortunately a real minority. Knowing who your real friends are is an invaluable lesson and I'm elated to know that I have a significant amount. People tend to treat you as you treat them, so if you're nice to them, they're nice to you. Few things give more assurance than the knowledge that there will be people always on your side in situations. What makes friendship is the knowledge that there is a person able to empathise with you in situations. Not being able to do so properly can just seem like you're selfishly trying to simplify things for yourself, hence what it really confirms is ignorance.

Integral to my development is never forgetting just how far along the road of recovery I have already come. It's all too easy to take things for granted and I am just far too British to be comfortable with praising myself, which seems overly Americanised and vulgar. One trait that has been endowed by me is the stiff-upper lip. What I still have is the desire to be renowned for something. This can negatively lead at times to me feeling that I am living my life against a clock.

Certainly my life seems back to front at times; I had always been an aspirational person from a very young age, as much as this warranted some satirising. In my early twenties I can already predict it to be unlikely that I will be faced with anything as dramatic as a TBI; it is far from impossible though. Things always having the potential to get worse, I'm just glad that I can now experience a life again that is enjoyable rather than just satisfactory. Meeting new people I don't any longer feel that I necessarily need to tell people of my experience; I'll only tell them if it happens to arise in conversation. In this respect control has now returned to me. I cannot overstate just how fortunate I feel to have the support of such a phenomenal family and group of friends; the amount of gratitude that I have is colossal. These things are uneasy to say as a Brit then it's difficult to feel that this is just something that you can genuinely say. As long as you've got a cluster of real mates in life, then you'll be alright.

13- You Really Got Me

The British Criminal Justice System is an institution that I have unfortunately come to have a real grievance towards. The process of bringing the perpetrators of my accident to court was inevitably a slow process. The male who (it would be easier if the evidence led me to think otherwise) was engaged in a race with the white Mitsubishi that struck us was found 'Not Guilty'. My natural bias is acknowledged by me, though I think the witness evidence given should have been compelling enough to force him to pay in some way for his crime. Speaking as a liberal an ex-juror; (who too found the defendant 'not guilty' due to lack of definitive evidence) I have a real gripe with the order in which British criminal trials are lead.

To me the fickleness of the general public draws obvious questions to the order in which trials are conducted, with the defendant unexceptionally giving their evidence last. What also antagonises me, are the people who feel justified in saying thinking that I must not recognise the full extent of how the criminal law works to feel so wounded. Cheated is a thing that I felt, particularly given that I was such a conformist individual; it has always seemed to make life simpler for me in many ways. In my mind the trial still appears to be a gross miscarriage of justice. Penal penalties largely rest on justification of punishment and this is loaded with disproportionality with the pain and suffering caused. Going with the populist position of being more punitive that the system in place is not something to which I adhere, though under the current system I feel that I've been unfairly victimised. Not that there is really ever such thing as being justifiably victimised.

The political spectrum divides people's reaction to the trial; most people seem to go somewhere in one of two ways. The right-wing group naturally just use this trial to express how the criminal justice system has clearly gone down the pan

71

(i.e. that the accused should have been 'hung, drawn and quartered'). Then there are the intellectual Left can say how no good can come out of punishment and they are the victim of unfair society blah de blah. I've always agreed with the latter camp, but then I always had an awful lot more faith in the British Criminal Justice system than I've been left with now.

The potential is still very much there with our legal system, but the legal performance of barristers seems incredibly ugly to me, aided by both their prescribed appearance and delusional ego. This is embarrassing in that this exaggerated persona frequently rides over somebody pathetic. Manipulating the truth so that guilty people can walk free in order to boost you own credence is certainly not something that I envy.

Yes I'll have to admit that the trial's close did induce me to have a bit of a tirade. I don't regret this. Believe me, I could have worded my outburst more 'eloquently' than I did; I'm still angered slightly that I was very much the exception here, rather than the norm. The Legal system clearly wants changing. If we had always acted towards things we disapprove of in the same way as many people did, I don't see how the emancipation of slavery would ever have been witnessed or that women would ever have attained the franchise. From my standpoint, this doesn't contradict my conformity at all because I try to make it quite lucid that conforming to society should simplify things for people. It was only down to complicated and convoluted procedure that allowed the trial to be finalised with a verdict of 'Not Guilty'.

When there are such profound failures of justice and do not comprehend how this is in my own or the Establishment's interest. Being officially commended on allowing people to evade responsibility is not something that I am at all comfortable with. Barristers can sometimes only be commiserated on the inadequacy of their at times, pathetic job. Resentful is something that I am of just accepting the verdict of the trial just based on the insufficiency of evidence. Wishing anything else seems rather primitive, though I can't help but feel let-down by the law.

The fact that the trial would have cost our nation an incredibly large sum of time and money leads me towards feeling that much of the legal system, particularly barristers are profiting off of the back of blood-money.

In fairness, the barrister who featured in my trial was doing no more than making a success of what was required of him by his profession. Whether I despise him or the system to which he is part of to a greater extent is something of a chicken and egg question I feel. Ultimately he was just doing his job, though as a functioning citizen within this system, I can no longer feel at all proud to be a part of it.

A fulfilled existence, it always comes down to overly taking for granted things that we already have, rather than what we may think that we're lacking; this is again where I'll recommend visiting the developing world. You appear to get dealt a pack of cards in life and to me it seems your duty to make the best of this. People could say that this is all too easy to say how lucky I am, perhaps so, but there certainly are a great deal of people lots more privileged that I have ever been.

Lamenting unlucky situations never gets you anywhere. This isn't down to fate, just general circumstances. Without wanting this to sound like any self-help book, we should all sometimes take the time to appreciate what we've got, rather than what we lack. We, I'm sure can all too easily think in excess of a billion excuses why things haven't necessarily always gone our way. Having used the example of getting dealt a pack of cards in life, though I'm incredibly uncomfortable is something that I am with the idea that everything is pre-ordained in terms of fate.

Nobody likes a sob-story and life's certainly not always fair for everyone. Worse is the idea that everything happens for a reason. This all seems rather like a simplistic way of trying to explain things. It is funny (in a way devoid of any wit) how believers always shy away from the use of fate to explain anything bad happened. Fate just seems like a simplistic way of describing conditions.

Talking of interpreting situations, survivor's guilt was something that I was initially far too ill to suffer from upon coming around from my coma. I wouldn't say that I have it too badly now, but I feel occasionally rather limited by feeling that I need to justify every passing second of my life to myself. As much as wanting to continue enjoying living life, I can't say that I'm particularly scared of death. Perhaps this is just far too easy to claim at my age, though our time will all come, so as with religion, I can't foresee it as worth wasting your precious existence on fretting over. Death's one of the final taboo's and this needs to change.

Personally I spend a significant amount of time contemplating death. This is not at all in a remotely morbid way, rather it is just a thing that I feel is rather ethereally cleansing. The irony is that I know that in thinking about death, there is nothing to really think about.

Can't we all just embrace the fact that there are things and resort to wanting, rather than needing to know that answer about certain things. Can't we just enjoy mystery without needing to fabricate answers as religion seems to have given everything.

Turning away from a culture and everything that it can offer to fulfil you always seems rather stupid to me. For me this frequently involves trips to public houses, restaurants, exhibitions and generally just being out and about. I'll be biased in terms of enjoying drinking, yet I've always renowned doing so as a fantastic way of breaking barriers meeting people. Socialising at public houses is rather conventional which seems to make frequenting pubs an easy way of earning some enjoyment. What we all must want is a place to converse with people socially in a relaxed atmosphere.

Occasionally people that beg to differ can sound rather infantile in expressing that they're 'too above' going to the pub it is often all too easy to counter with some inverted snobbery. In terms of entertaining opinions, I think that there is a fine line between people who you wish would voice their opinion more frequently and those who appear to do so just to antagonise. Apart from being pitiful, it would surely pay-off for both parties just to admit that you really know a great deal or just agree to differ on a particular subject.

Knowing that intelligence often has absolutely nothing to do with what side of an opinion you harbour just seems like part of getting used to adulthood. No matter how intelligent you are, there will always be more factual pieces of information that you don't yet have any awareness than things you concretely can ever be sure of unquestionably.

As I've come to increasingly understand the judicial system, I've come to conclude that there is nothing particularly exceptional about my trial. The thing that I can still have fury over concerns there being several cameras that would have been passed by the cars racing that had an absence of roll in them. One image of the cars would have been enough to ensure that a guilty verdict was reached. I know that there is no 100% proof that the driver on trial was involved with the accident; the evidence given lead me to believe that if he wasn't indeed the driver then I might as well believe in a religion.

If the speed cameras functioned as they ought, then a guilty verdict would have been reached instantaneously. The fact that the cameras not being correctly loaded with rolls of film highlights the fact that the trials close does nothing but broadcast the sloppiness residing within our justice and legal system.

There never seems to be a large quantity of space left for independence of thought or mind in the legal system. It is something understandable that consistency is imperative for the legal system to operate.

Excelling without our legal system depends upon not questioning many aspects of the procedures that you are undertaking and not questioning a system that you feel to be beneficial. This is certainly not to slate anybody that works within our current legal system; being a lawyer has never had any remote attraction

Emotions such as the stress felt at fervently having to revisit a meagre past experience is something that I feel aggrieved that the legal system seems to overlook when equating the compensatory sum to which you are entitled.

Restorative justice is something that I strongly advocate. There can never be anything at all healthy in a grudge, though letting go of this resentment is feeling incredibly testing. Confronting the Honda and Mitsubishi drivers with what they supposedly did and allowing them to recognise the suffering that they caused would I believe allow all of us to constructively move on with our lives. Increased difficulty is had by me, in terms of them not being found guilty by the system of racing, which I remain, convinced that they were. Bringing the beautiful old cliché I again, I'll try to forgive without ever forgetting.

14- Too Much Too Young

Living life one step at a time is a clichéd figure of speech that I have come to live by; principally because I've come to learn the hard way that nothing in life can ever be that definite. What nobody can ever prevent you from doing is attempting to enjoy yourself.

There should never be any long-lasting reason not to try and have a decent time. Repeating carpe diem, as I mentioned cornily in the preface, it is the only viable way in which to do this; it's rude not to. Often though as I find myself, it is all too easily said rather than done.

What I think I'm learning is just to try and take a step back and reassure yourself of how ridiculous the stuff you're often worrying about is. I'm a perpetual worrier who is now trying to learn not to; it's difficult because I've always known what a waste of both mine and other people's time. If you're a worrier too I'm sure that you'll understand the frustration of other people not understanding at all what it's like to worry. Oh how I'm jealous of them. It being presumed that you're engaged in worrying for the sake of it is incredibly exasperating, as it could not be further from the truth.

This goes along with me adhering to the belief that understanding is everything and if you do not, you become devoid of empathy. This has to be our most sophisticated emotion, being what supposedly separates us most from other species, as humans. There would surely be an awful lot of value to be gained on a joint account if our understanding of things was heightened. A problem shared is a problem halved, so I'm sure that us all having a greater understanding of each other would double the productivity universally. It has to be admitted that grateful, rather than guilty is something that I predominantly feel from being born in the Western World. It's unlikely that I could have survived a severe Brain Injury with it having occurred in the Developing World. You can completely appreciate situations without foreseeing that you can viably do anything to rectify them. This defeatist attitude lacks productivity.

It is probable that people do in fact have compassion for my accident in ways that I can sometimes fail to recognise. Conceivably it is not unnatural for me to feel at times like people have been rather unresponsive towards the circumstances of my situation. Overall though, this is not at all the case; in fact the polar-opposite.

Every episode of my life seems incredibly over-analysed and this has transcended to my judgements of myself. Occasionally people in caring professions seem to have a fervent propensity to feel that every element of life needs to be analysed. From my point of view, it really doesn't need to always be vocalised.

Often I think that perceptions of things are best kept to yourself, as it is not at all productive in anybody's interest to know. As a result, being asked to define you is never an easy task. Voicing my opinion on a particular issue just doesn't always seem necessary due to more than idleness on my-part. An extrovert is a label that I have been given. This is strange considering the degree of shyness I was born with and naturally still have under certain circumstances.

Again this statement will not make me popular, but to me shyness is a fundamental personality trait that we should all try and overcome; not doing so can make you appear rather narcissistic. This does indeed sound ruthless, though being honest I think that we can all say that it's uncomfortable being lumbered stuck next to the shy stranger at a restaurant or bar. As a shy little boy, I can remember what it feels like relying upon others to 'excuse' your shyness. It was reassuring being able to place the weight on others to account for you having being rude in not really engaging in conversation. The childishness of it speaks for itself.

The principal objective in life must be to enjoy yourself and shyness limits this so much, as you can appear merely to idiotically believe that some people aren't worthy of your company. Of course it is wrong to say that shyness is generally deliberate or something that humans can always exert a great deal of control over, though along with prudishness it can make somebody be appearing rather repressed.

Continuing with this senseless rant, it is all too easy for me to comprehend how such a quantity of intelligent people can be apolitical. Politics has the tendency to come across as highly complicated and it should never do; this is what must make it so broadly inaccessible. The idea that politics constitutes a discipline in its own right, rather than any analysis of societal procedure seems to be the forefront of the problem. A person sitting on the fence about everything just doesn't always make for engaging conversation. Regardless of whether you have any political affiliation, you must harbour opinions.

Saying all of this though, politics in itself always creeping into everyday conversation can be confrontational and unnecessary. There's usually something I find more fun to talk about. Everybody must have an opinion and it seems vital to be able to respect and acknowledge other people's opinion, without agreeing at all yourself. Having an apolitical opinion on everything can appear like segregating yourself from any unified society. For me, it is easier to feel more united with somebody staunchly opposed to you politically than somebody who never engages.

Voting is the singular chance our society gives of expressing yourself and if you want to abstain, it is surely better to spoil a ballot paper than not voice yourself at all. It is all too easy to detach yourself from society and it seems better to express disengagement, rather than do nothing about it. If you do nothing to formally express your interests, you sacrifice the right to moan.

Acting mute, when you can enjoy the option of having a voice seems pretty senseless. You can say "but my vote doesn't make any difference"; tough, you can't communicate with the country any other way. What you're really doing is divorcing yourself from society. It seems to me highly illogical not to be left-wing. From the mass perspective in the UK now, I doubt that anybody would be against the National Health

Service (NHS), though it seems that the NHS is taken for granted by everybody at the present. Selfishly people are glad of the things that left-wing parties may have done, yet refuse to pay anything extra for mutual benefit themselves. Conservatism just seems to slowdown progress. Being inflicted with a trauma you especially learn that that there is really no time to waste in regard to treatment and making improvements where it's needed.

Acceptance seems to me to be the most precious thing that you can gain in life; for both yourself and everybody else can only benefit from this. What accepting seems to do is overcome nervousness - it would be difficult to be a bigot if you had more understanding of alternative cultures - the alternative is to be afraid? People must be far more satisfied when they have a greater understanding of others, rather than compete with one another. This is one element that has been raised by me in terms of people suffering various disabilities. Take the handicap Multiple Sclerosis (MS) to illustrate how there is complete asymmetry between a person's physical and mental capacity.

It is more than aggravating to speculate upon how few people seem aware of this. This then ties-in with the shame of having potential difficulties; if you're too a proud person, you'll see how belittling it feels to have difficulty with regular tasks. It is often in therapy that there is a natural propensity to overprotect patients. It was found particularly hard, as living without too much restrictiveness has always been paramount to me. Hearing the disparaging sounding words, "well it's your choice," is a much more effective way that I'm glad my parents adopted of dissuading a family member or close friend from doing something. Close to a million times more likely of doing something is a thing that I'll confess that I am if I'm being "told" not to by somebody I don't respect. Making mistakes (take learning to ride a bike) is often the only method of learning.

People, who have not ever tried anything for themselves, can often seem venerably dull. In terms of trying to make you sound increasingly interesting for advertising having tried things solely for the sake of having tried them seems rather thoughtless to me. On this note, it seems highly illogical to want everything that you've ever done or tried to always want to be broadcast.

Learning how to master being selective about your company and who to relate certain pieces of information to just seems like part of an educated adulthood. To me, it does just feel incredibly satisfying and inclusive when I know that I have already experienced some of the topics of other people's conversation. Equally there is no reason to ever feel sidelined for never having tried things that other people have. You have to appreciate those significant elements of your lifestyle may create discomfort if related to other people. Part of maturity is gauging how pieces of information shall be received by certain audiences, or just being beyond caring.

Superficiality is unbearable. I too am capable of making shallow comments, though I'll claim that this is justifiable based on the fact that I know how idiotic these remarks are. Whatever organisations you belong to, there always seem to be clusters of incredibly phoney people. They pose around and make irrelevant remarks and are always swarming around with whatever of their 'crises' that having been born with a silver-spoon in their mouth always allows them to possess.

The saddest thing is that they never seem to have any genuine associates, as they're all too consumed with their deluded image to ever have any real friends, as everybody in their 'circle' just bitches about one another to each other. Ultimately they just have so much insecurity and just come to be overly reliant on their delusional image. To me, they are always too repugnant to ever exude anything remotely attractive. Effort is the main thing that is required to be their real friends. Individually these people are always nice and decent company, it is just that together they are a swarm, like pack animals, that it is incredibly tiring to be around. I'll admit it now, there was once a time when this is a mould that I had some jealousy of; I'd even be convinced that my gripes with their pretentious lifestyle were envy. There maybe even was a time when trying to emulate this was something that I tried;

thankfully that time's long passed. If it's just down to the fact that I could never quite cut the mould. Maybe this is because I was never cool enough to form a real part of this group, I'm so grateful. Instrumentality people are all alright, it's just that these flocks occupied by everybody's self-interests are tiring.

Using young age-old wisdom, just being nice and treating people as you would like to be treated tends to work successfully in this life. To me this has involved outgrowing a stage where everything relates to each individual's status and just having faith with your own position in life. Ultimately it has resulted in me being left to handle yet another paradox left by the accident. I am confronted with concurrently feeling like I have been left behind many of my contemporaries in terms of establishing myself. Whilst this has been said I feel that I could never have attained my supposed level of maturity without this having happened. No matter how much certain things go beyond any generation gap, (which is largely artificial in itself) there are certain life experiences that you have to which only people of your generation can remotely relate. Regardless of to what extent you attempt to imagine or remember what it's like to be of a certain age, without actually being at that point, your interpretation will always be rather flawed.

Talking as an overly introspective person at the best of times and fail to properly comprehend being otherwise. Like everything the merits of this outlook are grounded on a fine-line that it is difficult not to cross, between being unconstructively hyper-analytical and just unconscious towards your environment. Like everything else in life, perfection is grounded on a healthy-balance that is just impossible to ever find.

5- All I really want To Do

Making my account of enduring a Brain Injury personal to you is something which I hope that I've achieved. My prolonged ordeal of having a Brain Injury is now an experience that I will never shed and would feel largely incomplete without. So as already stated, from my experience you need to deal with the cards that you get thrown and make the best of good and bad circumstances. Without wishing to sound sanctimonious, we all need to be prepared to take the positive and negative experiences of life as an integral part of being human. Without sounding too holier than thou!

When I was a child, I was convinced that all was accessible. I'd have a successful career, so be rich and probably famous by now. Without being depressive, part of adulthood is learning that pipe-dreams aren't always attainable, though I'm just adamant that we have to always cling to our aspirations to healthily get through life. Not being overly definite about anything is something that I've found to be key.

Statistically speaking I've already lived around a third of my life and this is something that I find unbelievable. I'm convinced that internally you never should feel aged, despite how many years you've got to your name. The general thought-process that exists within me has never seemed to alter and this is something that I think is probably the same for everyone.

I just wish that everybody were able to relish life.

This fulfilment of life can only really be achieved by being surrounded by people who are also game to make the best of things and enjoy themselves. We only live once so I think that you're cheating yourself and others by refusing to do so. What's been found integral to me is re-carving my identity amongst both family and peers. One of the most reassuring things to me is that people have volunteered in coming forward to declare how evident it is that nothing about me beyond the voice and physicality has changed.

Feeling that I've not had to mould a new identity amongst people that know me has been a welcome relief. More assuring still is the fact that I know that I've always been well aware that no morsel of my personality has changed.

Sometimes I wish that people would give more thought before making such declarations estimating my characteristics to others, as it's an incredibly penetrating conversation matter. With this in mind I have full-confidence in myself again and am able to completely trust my own judgement as much as I ever could. Certainly it never feels indebted by me to necessarily ever divulge my experience to acquaintances that I may not have seen for a number of years.

Revelling in my existence being able to still persist in a way that I am comfortable with is the ultimate confirmation that life's back under my control. The experiences of having endured a Brain Injury shall be everlasting, but they can now be a secondary aspect of my life.

There are such magnitudes of things that I have been through having a Brain Injury that I shall never fully detach myself from. Being a realist, there is no choice whatsoever about this aspect of life. It all comes back to, "making the best of circumstances," and it would seem ludicrous to waste energy doing anything else.

At first I was overly defensive, particularly on returning to academia upon accepting that any changes had been made on account of having been inflicted with a TBI. Now I can appreciate the elements of myself that have altered, without having the need to prove anything to anybody.

It has already been confirmed that nothing has altered remotely in terms of my quintessence, so I am able to take on board adaptations to confront the incredibly subtle differences to my functioning. Having been inflicted with a TBI is certainly no longer a predominant part of my life and this is something that has now been firmly established. From an individual perspective, life is invaluable to myself, though it's been found predominantly reassuring by me is to know that the world will continue to go around and around long indifferent to my existence.

The experience of having a Brain Injury is not something that can ever be walked away from, but the choice over who are divulged things has been reclaimed and this triumph shall never voluntarily be sacrificed. It can very much now take a back seat in comparison to the primary focus being to living my life best possible. If there is one thing that this entire ethos has taught me, it's to try and allow yourself and others to enjoy life as best as possible, as there is no other worthwhile reward to be searching.

The recovery process that I am going through never feels as though it shall end as you are surely ever absorbing new pieces of information and improving yourself. As long as you treat others as you would like to be treated yourself, all should go pretty smoothly.

Like many elements of my vision of an idealised life, this really does seem to be geared towards a mutual benefit. Perhaps it is too much of a foolhardy thing to say, but it would be pretty difficult for me to be socially embarrassed these days given all the traumatic experiences that I've felt myself to be going through. It was always felt by me that almost however enjoyable a time that I was having, the grass was bound to always be greener somewhere else. Perhaps this can be seen as a disturbing thing to say at any age, but if I were to perish tomorrow, I think that I could say that I had certainly fully enjoyed living my life.

Although I will never be fully compensated for what has been incurred by me, you can never seemingly do much other than take whatever positive that can be extracted from the negative. I feel autonomous to a degree that far exceeds what I believe myself ever capable of reaching prior to my accident occurring. By no means has the accident reduced my quality of life; if anything it has increased my confidence. Reserved is not something I ever felt I ever was particularly, but now I feel that the ability to effortlessly induce acquaintances to open-up about anything. This is incredibly liberating and further goes towards me feeling that my Brain Injury has earned me an increased amount of social freedom. Now, I can class my Brain Injury as an instrumentally definitive episode of my life, rather than something through which I'm defined. Inner-peace is something which I feel that I've finally reached.

Having graduated with a 2:1 from the glorious university of York in English and Politics post-morbidly, I can confidently say that a bleak prognosis is something that it is all too possible to turn around. Relief and triumph are the emotions that I predominantly feel. The degree outcome that I have attained is far from anything inferior to any of my aspirations prior to being brain-damaged.

Shit can certainly hit the fan around any corner and at any point is this life. Sadly we have absolutely no say over trouble coming to us, although you can orchestrate how you deal with it happening. The great family and group of friends that I have surrounding me have made my recovery easier.

Determination and perseverance is all that you need. As long we don't take each other too seriously then life seems to be enjoyable enough.